AF657077

Highlights on
PHARMACOVIGILANCE

P G Yeole
Dhanalakshmi Iyer
Institute of Pharmaceutical Education & Research
Wardha (M.S.)-442001

2013

Studium Press (India) Pvt. Ltd.

Highlights on PHARMACOVIGILANCE

© 2013

This book contains information obtained from authentic and highly regarded sources. Reprinted material is quoted with one acknowledgement, and sources are indicated. A wide variety of references are listed. Reasonable efforts have been made to publish reliable data and information. The opinion expressed in the book is largely of the contributors. The publisher and authors disclaim any liability, in whole or in part, arising from information contained in the publication or for the consequences of their use.

All rights are reserved under International and Pan-American Copyright Conventions. Apart from any fair dealing for the purpose of private study, research, criticism or review, as permitted under the Copyright Act, 1956, no part of this publication may be reproduced, stored in a retrieval system or transmitted, in any form or by any means–electronic, electrical, chemical, mechanical, optical, photocopying, recording or otherwise–without the prior permission of the copyright owner.

ISBN: 978-93-80012-59-9

Published by:

Studium Press (India) Pvt. Ltd.
4735/22, 2nd Floor, Prakash Deep Building (Near PNB),
Ansari Road, Darya Ganj, New Delhi-110002
Phone: +91-11-43240200-15 (15 lines); Fax: +91-11-43240215
jngovil@gmail.com; jngovil@hotmail.com

Printed at:

Akash Press, New Delhi

Foreword

The government of a country plays an important role in decision making process with regards to the development and evolution of pharmacovigilance. The developed countries like United States, Japan and European Union which have the largest pharmaceutical market, have evolved stringent regulations for drug safety measures. Even the regulatory authorities in many developing countries have framed regulations and guidelines for pharmacovigilance. The non-compliance of these regulations leads to severe disciplinary action against the offenders.

A well laid pharmacovigilance system is essential for any pharmaceutical company. The pharmaceutical manufacturers are also required to adhere to and comply with local regulations of the country, where the product holds marketing authorization. The regulatory authorities, pharmaceutical industries, academia and health care professionals are to be geared up for induction of necessary strategic changes in order to make the pharmaceutical world hazard-free. The progress is expected in the arena of signal detection, risk-benefit evaluations and in taking appropriate actions to mitigate avoidable risks to the patients. The adverse drug reactions are required to be collected and subjected to risk-benefit analysis.

For pharmacovigilance to achieve the highest standards there must be an attitude of zero tolerance when it comes to compromising on patient safety. The importance of pharmacovigilance in a country will grow with growing awareness amongst the public. This book is thus, a step towards generating awareness particularly, amongst the student population who can get the necessary know-how about pharmacovigilance, before they take a plunge into the professional world. Important nuances pertaining to pharmacovigilance such as, ADRs, MeDRA, PSURs, signal detection, safety data bases, ADRs, pharmacoepidemiology, regulations, etc. have been discussed thoroughly in this book. The text of the book reflects upon different facets of pharmacovigilance, which are easy to understand. The information provided in the text of the book is useful for the readers from different backgrounds to understand fundamental and comprehensive aspects of drug safety. The authors, Dr. P.G.Yeole and Dr. D.Iyer, have expressed the subject matter in a very lucid manner enabling readers from diverse fields viz. regulators, pharmaceutical and biotech companies, pharmacovigilators, medical and paramedical professionals to find ready reference to a specific topic. regarding pharmacovigilance *per se.*

This piece of information will be useful in strengthening the drug safety aspects in the health-care domain of our country.

Prof. (Dr.) C.K. Kokate
Vice-Chancellor
KLE University
Belgaum

Preface

The awareness related to growth and potential of pharmacovigilance as a significant discipline of medicine has become very necessary. Understanding the need of the hour pertaining to safety aspects of a drug in market, the book: "Highlights of Pharmacovigilance" has been penned down.

Pharmacovigilance and all drug safety issues are relevant for everyone whose life is touched in any way by medical interventions. Having said this, it then becomes quite significant to put in painstaking efforts to meet the challenges that lie ahead in the next ten years. To make sure that pharmacovigilance bring along with it full benefits, milestones have to be achieved. Pros and cons of the existing system have to be critically inspected to make deliberate and calculated decisions. Collaboration, communication at local, regional and international levels, has to be seriously taken up so that pharmacovigilance delivers its full benefits.

Thus the book is an attempt to make every reader aware of the fundamentals of pharmacovigilance, an in-depth of the common jargons associated with pharmacovigilance, the initiatives by various bodies viz: ICH, WHO, CIOMS for bettering the pharmacovigilance structure. Further the book also highlights specific aspects pertaining to MedDRA®, Periodic safety Update Reports (PSURs) and SUSARS, basics of Pharmacoeconomics, Pharacoepidemiology etc.

The readership would extend to the following groups of people:

- Policy makers at all levels of healthcare, particularly those concerned with drug policy
- Staff and consultants in national drug regulatory authorities
- Healthcare practitioners including doctors, nurses and pharmacists
- Pharmaceutical industry executives and scientists
- Professional staff in national pharmacovigilance centers

- Editors of medical and scientific journals
- Health epidemiologists
- Health economists
- Professional staff of poison and drug information centers
- Health administrators
- Consumer groups and patient support groups
- Legal advisors in health care
- Schools of health sciences, and
- The concerned layperson.

This work has been possible by the grace of the all prevailing Almighty and is indebted to Him. Also, in presenting this piece of work, we would like to acknowledge all our well-wishers and friends who were instrumental in rendering the intellectual stimuli and unstinted support in every stage of drafting this book.

Acknowledgements

This work has been possible by the grace of the all prevailing Almighty and is indebted to Him. We also extend our heartfelt thanks to all our well wishers and friends and associates who have directly or indirectly been instrumental in this piece of work. Thank you readers....

P G Yeole

Dhanalakshmi Iyer

About the Authors

Dr. P G Yeole

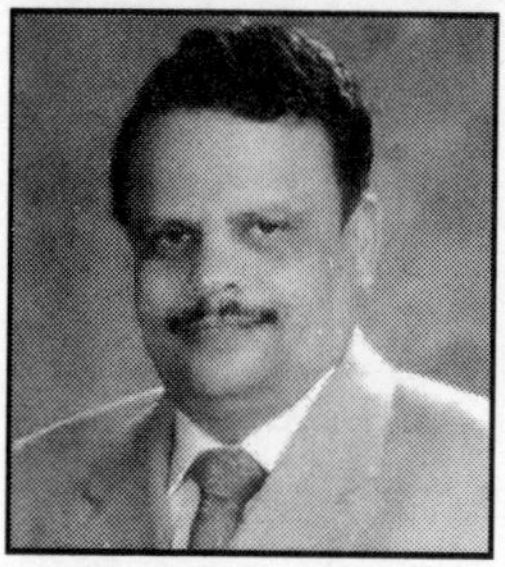

Prof. (Dr.) P.G. Yeole, a Professor and Principal at Institute of Pharmaceutical Education and Research, Wardha (M.S.) India, has over 3 decades experience in academia and has earned his Ph.D. from Nagpur University. Currently, a dean of Faculty of medicine of R.T.M. Nagpur University, he was also a member of Management Council, academic council and senate of Rastrasant Tukdoji Maharaj Nagpur University, Nagpur. Besides these, he has also multi-tasked various functions by being a chairman of the Board of studies of Pharmaceutical sciences of Nagpur University and a member of Board of studies in Pharmaceutical sciences in various universities of India. A compilation of around 51 publications in reputed pharmaceutical journals is yet another acclaim to his accomplishments. He has supervised 14 Ph.D. and 55 M.Pharm candidates. Dr. Yeole is a President of Association of Pharmaceutical Teachers of India. He has been emphatically working for the cause of up-liftment of pharmacy profession in India by being associated with different National and International professional societies. His immense contribution to the profession of Pharmacy in India is honored by bestowing on him esteemed state and national academic awards.

Dr. Dhanlakshmi Iyer

Dr. D. Iyer, has worked with Academia and Industry alike with an experience of over 12 years now. She has worked with Drug Safety, Regulatory Affairs and Medical writing domains of Pharmaceutical Multinationals. An Associate Professor, at Institute of Pharmaceutical

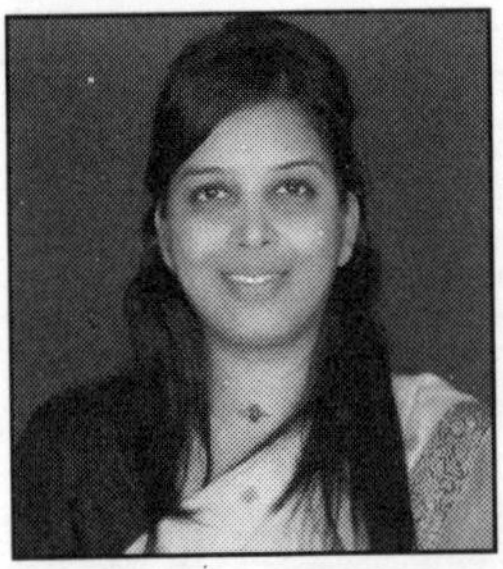

Education and Research, Wardha, she has guided six M. Pharm candidates at Nagpur University. Dr. Iyer has also been actively involved in various Research and Industrial Projects of Pharmaceutical and Herbal Companies. She functions as an Intellectual Property Consultant offering wide range consultation in the area of Patents, Trademarks, Geographical Indications, Copyrights and Industrial Designs. She has been a guest speaker to various National and International Forums/ Conventions, and has around 10 publications to her credit.

Table of Contents

1

Introduction to Pharmacovigilance

Clinical research and pharmacovigilance have come a long way since the thalidomide disaster. The disaster alerted the world regarding safety issues pertaining to the drug and triggered a wave of governmental and regulatory activities in the 1960's which defined the principles of modern clinical research and pharmacovigilance. Thalidomide was introduced in 1957 and widely prescribed as an allegedly harmless treatment for morning sickness and nausea. Within a short span, it was linked to a congenital anomaly which caused severe birth defects (Fig. 1) in children of women who had been prescribed this medicine during pregnancy. By 1965, thalidomide was removed from the market in many countries. Systems were developed for the collection of individual case histories of Adverse Drug Reactions (ADRs) and evaluation of them. The collection of international ADR reports in a central database would serve the important function of helping national drug regulatory authorities, improving the safety profile of medicines and assistance in avoiding further disasters.

Several disasters led to an awareness that drugs not only can heal but also can harm including sudden death caused by chloroform anaesthesia in 1877 and fatal hepatic necrosis due to arsenicals in 1922. In the United States a tragic mistake in the formulation of a children's syrup in the late 1930s was the trigger for setting up the product authorization system under the Food and Drug Administration (FDA). FDA had the authority to review new drugs for safety, by scrutinizing animal studies and small human volunteer trials for any signs of serious hazards. Child deaths after diethylenglycol was mistakenly used to solubilise sulphanilamides in 1937 led to the first enactment of legislation on adverse reactions Federal Food, Drug and Cosmetic Act, 1938 (FFDA) as mentioned in Table 1.

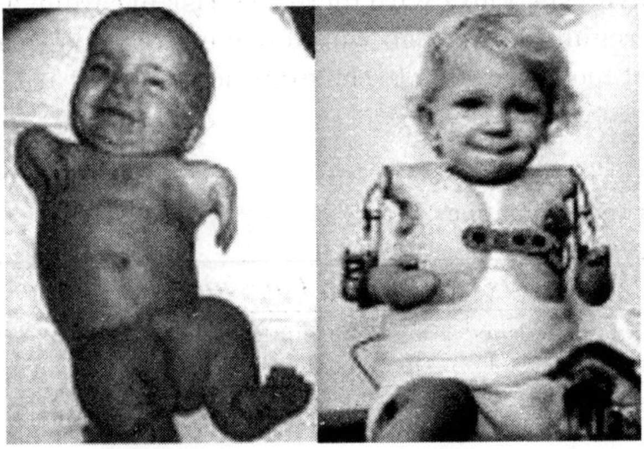

Fig. 1: Birth defects observed in children following the Thalidomide Disaster

Following 100 deaths in France in 1952 after diethyl tin diodide and the thalidomide tragedy of the 1960s, in England and in Germany with reports of foetal abnormalities (phocomelia and micromelia) in relation with the use of a new sleep-inducing thalidomide, there was a rapid increase in laws, regulations and guidelines for reporting and evaluating the data on safety, quality and efficacy of new medicinal products. In the summer of 1962 a new bill amending the 1938 Food, Drug and Cosmetic Act (FDCA), the Kefauver-Harris Amendments, gave the FDA the power to approve or disallow the introduction of new drugs and the continued marketing of established compounds based on substantial evidence of their therapeutic efficacy as well as safety. Around 1980 it became compulsory to record side effects (adverse drug reactions) by the regulatory authorities in many countries to allow for a continual monitoring of the risk and benefit of products both in the investigational phase before authorization and as postmarketing surveillance when the product is commercialised as an authorized product. The consequences of this are that over the last 30 years there have been continued instances of drug recalls or precautionary statements due to the discovery of potential hazards during their use, some more notable examples include:

practolol and the mucocutaneous syndrome, benoxaprofen and hepatic disorders/deaths in the elderly, temafloxacin and haemolytic anaemia, fenfluramine/phenteramine and valvulopathy or pulmonary hypertension, terfenadine or cisapride and potential cardiac arrhythmias (especially in association with interacting agents), cerivastatin (Lipobay) and rhabdomyolysis, Vioxx with increased risk of cardiovascular events. The various regulations which were enacted due to a series of adverse reactions that took place due to consumption of drugs are listed in Table 1 below.

Table 1: Laws and Regulations

	Key events resulting in Laws and Regulations
1820	Physicians concerned about the quality of domestic and imported drugs convened the first U.S. Pharmacopeia (USP) convention. This convention wrote guidelines for the formulation of drug products, resulting in the publication of the U.S.P. which contains information about drugs including source, physical and chemical properties, tests for purity and identify, assay method of storage, category and dosage.
1848	The Import Drugs Act of 1848 allowed U.S. Customs officials to inspect shipments of imported drugs. This function was later assumed by federal agents of the Bureau of Chemistry (renamed the FDA in 1930).
1877	Sudden death caused by chloroform anaesthesia 1898. The Bayer Company sold heroin as "a superior cough suppressant".
1906	Pure Food and Drugs Act of 1906: Problems with medicines and foods outraged the public and Congress. Required manufacturers to list ingredients contained in their products, meet standards of strength and purity established in the U.S.P. Amended over next 30 years to make labelling drugs with false claims a crime and to require physicians to have a license number to prescribe narcotics.
1911	In Germany evaluation of marketed medicines was the responsibility of the Congress of Internal Medicine later known as Medicines Commission of the German Medical Profession (AkdÄ).
1922	Fatal hepatic necrosis due to arsenicals.
1938	Federal Food, Drug and Cosmetic Act of 1938 following the manufacturer of sulfanilamide tablets, a popular cold remedy, with a more palatable liquid version, with a sweet raspberry taste. It turned out that the compound used to dissolve the tablets into solution was diethylene glycol, a deadly poison related to antifreeze. The FDC Act required proof of safety before a new drug could be marketed in the New Drug Application, allowed prosecution for

Table 1: *(Contd...)*

Table 1: *(Contd...)*

	Key events resulting in Laws and Regulations
	false claims of drugs, without having to prove intent to defraud, OTC but not prescription drugs, had to be labelled with adequate warnings and directions for use. The beginning of federal regulations governing the drug development and approval process (CFR).
1951	The Durham-Humphrey Amendment required certain drugs to be available only through a prescription from a licensed physician.
1952	In France, sudden deaths after diethyl tin diodide was mistakenly used in a skin preparation.
1958 & 1961	In Germany the Medicines Commission German Medical Profession (Arzneimittelkommission der deutschen Ärzteschaft) now Scientific Expert Committee of the German Medical Association reinforce request for the submission of adverse drug reactions following thalidomide birth defect tragedy (Adverse drug reaction form introduced in 1963 and forwarded to Federal Board of Health).
1961	First German Medicines Act with reform of public health including pharmacovigilance in 1978.
1962	Kefauver-Harris Drug Amendment of Federal Food, Drug and Cosmetic Act of 1938 was introduced following the thalidomide birth defect tragedy. Although not licensed in USA the FDA discovered that 2.5 million tablets of thalidomide were distributed to 1,270 U.S. physicians as samples. 200,000 American patients received thalidomide. The amendment required drugs to be proven effective as well as safe prior to marketing, required drug companies to register with the FDA, and gave FDA "explicit authority to require compliance with good manufacturing practices.
1966	FDA released the Guidelines for Reproduction Studies/WHO.
1968	WHO Programme for International Drug Monitoring now co-ordinated by the Uppsala Monitoring Centre.
1974	National Research Act of 1974 (45 CFR 46): The National Commission for the Protection of Human the Protection of Human Subjects in Biomedical and Subjects in Biomedical: Investigational Review Board/ Ethics Committee.
1979	The Belmont Report from National Commission: Respect for Perrsons, Beneficence, Justice
1990	International Conference on Harmonisation (ICH) Guidelines.
1991	Common Rule (Investigational Review Board, Informed consent, Selection of Patients)

World Health Organization (WHO) and Pharmacovigilance

As discussed earlier, the disaster that followed thalidomide in 1961 brought up a need to regulate pharmacovigilance not only by the national competent (regulatory) authorities but also over and above this at an international level in 1963 adopted a resolution stressing the need for early action in regard to dissemination of information on adverse drug reactions was adopted in the Sixteenth World Health Assembly. This further led to initiation of the WHO Pilot Research Project for International Drug Monitoring in 1968. The purpose of this was to develop a system, applicable internationally, for detecting previously unknown or poorly understood adverse effects of medicines forming the basis of the practice and science of pharmacovigilance to improve the safe and cost-effective use of medicines by avoiding further disasters in both developed and developing countries in the interests of improved public health. The 1968, International Pilot Programme was followed by the WHO Programme for International Drug Monitoring which is now co-ordinated by the Uppsala Monitoring Centre (UMC) in Uppsala, Sweden, under the supervision of an international board. The principal function of the Uppsala Monitoring Centre is to manage the international database of adverse drug reaction reports received from participating countries. The Programme includes more than sixty countries with active participation of regional reporting centres (housed within hospitals), interest groups, dedicated internal medicine and pharmacology department units, drug and poison information centres and other non-governmental organizations. As representatives from Germany, the Medicines Commission of the German Medical Profession has participated in the UMC since 1968. The introduction of Pharmacovigilance formally into the research and academic world, and its increasing integration into clinical practice occurred in the year 1992. This was due to the International Society of Pharmacoepidemiology (ISPE) in 1984 and of the European Society of Pharmacovigilance (ESOP –later ISoP–the International Society). Also execution of active surveillance systems to collect epidemiological information on adverse reactions to specific drugs was done by many countries.

Examples of such systems are:

- Prescription event monitoring systems (PEM) in New Zealand and UK

- Record linkage systems in the United States of America and Canada
- Case control studies in the United States of America.

The Council for International Organisations of Medical Sciences (CIOMS), an international, nongovernmental, non-profit organisation was established in 1949 by World Health Organisation (WHO) and the United Nations Educational, Scientific and Cultural Organisation (UNESCO). CIOMS in close collaboration with the WHO, launched its programme on drug development and use in the early 1980s. Suggestions and information on new developments in biology and medicine is assimilated and disseminated. It was decided that CIOMS shall provide an independent forum and facilitate discussions between national regulatory authorities and pharmaceutical companies on policy matters. CIOMS group is limited between 20–30 and consists of pharmacovigilance specialists from regulatory agencies and pharmaceutical manufacturers mainly from North America and Europe. Each working group is co-chaired by a member from a regulatory agency and a pharmaceutical manufacturer. Win Castle co-chaired all the working groups until her retirement in 2000. Every initiative mentioned below was completed successfully with her determination and hard work. As the CIOMS working groups have no legal jurisdiction, reliance is placed on other bodies to incorporate the CIOMS recommendations and guidelines into a regulatory or legislative framework.

There are various working groups of CIOMS based on the several initiatives being taken; Periodic Updates Safety Report (PSUR) is one such working group. There are also other working groups like CIOMS I, IA, II, III, IV, V, VI which takes various initiatives. CIOMS I deals with expedited reporting, CIOMS IA deals with data elements for electronic reporting, CIOMS II handles PSURs, CIOMS III with core clinical safety information, CIOMS IV takes care of benefit risk assessment, CIOMS V deals with post approval safety data management, CIOMS VI handles management of safety information from clinical trials.

The various activities undertaken by the CIOMS group is detailed below:

Expedited reporting: By CIOMS I was undertaken with a view to enable manufacturers report postmarketing ADRs with regards to a drug via an internationally acceptable method in a rapid, efficient and effective manner to the regulatory bodies.

CIOMS working group set the following criteria for expedited reporting of a foreign ADR:

1. Serious
2. Medically substantiated
3. Unexpected
4. Suspected *i.e.* related to the drug administered
5. Related to a product postmarketing
6. ADR occurrence in a identifiable patient

Electronic reporting: By CIOMS IA, laid emphasis on electronic reporting rather than paper work. The reports had to be submitted in a shared single database which could be accessed by all regulatory bodies and had restricted access to the manufacturers. This in turn would increase the time available for assessment of individual case studies and signal detection.

Periodic safety updates: By CIOMS II, commenced in the year 1989, was initiated with a view to reduce the chaos and disorder caused by requirement of different formats and time intervals for periodic safety update report submissions. Each individual local regulatory authority required varying periodic safety updates which was made more complex and difficult because of the varying due dates that was determined by the national licensing approval date which varied amongst different formulations of the same Active Pharmaceutical Ingredient (API). Thus to reduce the pressure on the manufacturers, it was decided by CIOMS II working group on a harmonized approach to PSURs submission.

It was recommended by the CIOMS II, that the PSUR must contain the following sections:

1. Introduction
2. Core data sheet–the reference document for determining expectedness *i.e.* was the adverse event related to a product expected.
3. Drugs' licensed status
4. Update on regulatory or manufacturers action taken for safety reasons.
5. Patient exposure
6. Individual case histories (CIOMS line listing)

7. Studies which would include targeted studies, newly analysed studies, published safety studies.
8. Overall safety evaluation
9. Important information after data lock point (DLP)

In addition, CIOMS line listings consist of the following features:

1. Company reference number
2. Country of origin of report
3. Source of report
4. Age of patient
5. Sex of patient
6. Dose of drug
7. Duration of treatment prior to event
8. Description of event
9. Outcome

Core clinical safety information (CCSI): An initiative by CIOMS III, the core clinical safety information is a document that clearly mentions the ADRs pertaining to a drug product. It sets out the minimum essential safety information by the manufacturer regarding a drug product. Care is taken to include only well established safety information in the CCSI. This reference document gives one an insight regarding the listedness and unlistedness of a product. This thus helps in making better informed decisions regarding consumption of a drug for a diseased condition.

Benefit risk evaluation: CIOMS IV working group deals with the benefit risk evaluation of a marketed product. It helps by providing guidelines to the regulators and manufacturers to assess the safety aspect of a product in its entirety by weighing the benefits and also the risks pertaining to a product, by taking into consideration the newly found (suspected or established) adverse event.

Good case management and reporting practices: This initiative of CIOMS V deals with aspects such as sources of individual case reports, Good case management practices, Good summary reporting practices, population exposure data, and worldwide clinical safety reporting regulations.

Management of safety information from clinical trials: Detecting safety signals pertaining to a suspected drug post marketing forms one major and significant aspect of pharmacovigilance studies. This is very important since till the time the new drug was tested for clinical trials, it was conducted for a limited population, limited duration of time, in unreal situations more often and also some special sensitive populations are generally not taken into consideration *i.e.* pediatric, geriatrics and pregnant women. Because of such limitations that are confronted premarketing of a new product, there are many instances and cases of adverse reactions which are suspected to have been caused due to the drug, that happens postmarketing during usage of these medications by patients in real life situations. Thus the differences between the premarketing, clinical trials conducted and postmarketing studies needs to be bridged. CIOMS VI enables conducting pharmacovigilance in a much better way from the development stage to post approval. A better approach of conducting clinical trials, to manage safety information in a more efficient way is initiated by CIOMS VI. This practical approach thus helps minimizing risks to an extent in the post approval marketing stage of the product. Thus the sixth CIOMS working group addressed the collection, monitoring, analysis, evaluation and overall management of safety information from clinical trials.

An opportunity was thus offered by CIOMS for policy makers, pharmaceutical manufacturers, government officials and academics to make recommendations on the communication of safety information between regulators and the pharmaceutical industry. The adoption of many of the recommendations of CIOMS by the International Conference on Harmonization (ICH) in the 1990s has had a notable impact on international drug regulation. The regulations that had to be catered to by the Manufacturing Authorisation Holder (MAH) along with various CIOMS initiatives is given in Table 2. 53 guidelines being published for quality, safety and efficacy by ICH has made its role exceptionally significant in the area of Pharmacovigilance. Thus it is very important on the part of a pharmacovigilator to know more about ICH, its inception, aim and contribution in the area of drug safety.

ICH was set up with a view of harmonisation in the following five categories:

1. New types of medicinal products

Table 2: Safety regulations for manufacturing authorisation holder

Pharmacovigilance: Regulations for Manufacturing Authorisation Holder
E2A CPMP/ICH/377/95 Clinical Safety Data Management: Definitions and Standards for Expedited Reporting
E2BM CPMP/ICH/287/95 Data Elements for Transmission of Individual Case Safety Reports (ICSR) (2002).
E2B (M) Data Elements for Transmission of ICSR (2004 Q & A)
E2B/M2 Maintenance of the Clinical Safety Data Management including the Maintenance of the Electronic Transmission of ICSR Message Specification
E2C CPMP/ICH/288/95 Clinical Safety Data Management: Periodic Safety Update Reports for Marketed Drugs. Addendum E2 C2004
E2D CPMP/ICH/4679/02 Post-Approval Safety Data Management: Definitions and Standards for Expedited Reporting ICH July 2003–draft guidance
E2E Pharmacovigilance Planning (PvP) ICH November 2003–draft guidance
CIOMS Working Group 1 International Reporting of Adverse Drug Reactions (CIOMS I Form)–served as a model for the development of the ICH Guideline E2A
CIOMS Working Group II International Reporting of Periodic Drug-Safety Update Summaries
PSUR format, content and frequency, which has been adopted by many regulatory authorities served as a model for the development the ICH Guideline E2C (addendum to ICH E2C from CIOMS WG V)
CIOMS Working Group III Guidelines for preparing Core Clinical-Safety Information (CCSI)
CIOMS Working Group III & V Guidelines for preparing Development Core Safety Information in preapproval environment (DCSI)
CIOMS Working Group IV Benefit-Risk Balance for Marketed Drugs. Evaluating Safety Signals
CIOMS Working Group V Current Challenges in Pharmacovigilance: Pragmatic Approaches
CIOMS Working Group VI Management of Safety Information from Clinical Trials
Volume 9–Pharmacovigilance Eudralex: Rules Governing Medicinal Products in the European Union
CPMP/PhVWP/108/99 Notice to Marketing Authorisation Holders Pharmacovigilance Guidelines now included in Eudralex Volume 9
CPMP/PhVWP/1618/01 Position Paper on Compliance with Pharmacovigilance Regulatory
Obligations Jan. 2002 (EMEA Inspections)
CPMP/ICH/3945/03 Post-Approval Safety Data Management–Definitions and Standards for Expedited Reporting
Directive 2001/83/EG Article 103 Now includied in Eudralex Vol. 1 'Qualified' Person responsible for pharmacovigilance.

2. Lack of harmonisation of current technical requirements
3. Shift to technically advanced and improved testing procedures.
4. Review of existing ICH guidelines resulting in major changes
5. Maintenance of existing ICH guidelines requiring minor changes.

ICH includes six parties *i.e.* authorities and associations of the three regions, *viz*: European Union, Japan and United States of America. The six parties are listed below:

1. The European Federation of Pharmaceutical Industries and Associations (EFPIA).
2. The Ministry of Health, Labour and Welfare of Japan (MHLW)
3. The Japanese Pharmaceutical Manuacturers Association (JPMA)
4. The European Commission representing the 25 member states of EU
5. The US Food and Drug Administration (FDA)
6. The Pharmaceutical Research and Manufaturers of America (PhRMA)

The ICH process is administered by the ICH steering committee and supported by the ICH secretariat that is run by the International federation of Pharmaceutical Manufacturers' Associations (IFMA) based out of Geneva. The ICH SC consists of two voting members from each ICH party, one non-voting member from IFPMA and one non-voting observer from each ICH observer party. The ICH SC also comprises a subcommittee, the ICH Global Cooperation Group (GCG), which is set up from one representative from each ICH party, the ICH Secretariat, WHO, EFTA, Health Canada and from five regional harmonisation initiatives, namely the Asian-Pacific Economic Cooperation (APEC), the Association of Southeast Asian Nations (ASEAN), the Gulf Cooperation Countries (GCC), the Pan-American Network on Drug Regulatory Harmonization (PANDRH) and the South African Development Community (SADC).

The development of an ICH guidelines/ recommendations is a process of five steps:

ICH STEP 1: DEVELOPMENT OF DRAFT CONSENSUS ICH GUIDELINE OR RECOMMENDATIONS

The ICH Expert Working Group (ICH EWG) develops the draft agreement ICH guideline or recommendations within a span of 2 years. The ICH Topic Leaders consult the proposals within the so-called 'Contact Network' of experts that each party has established within their regions and organisations for their scientific point of view with regards the draft consensus, to ensure that they reflect the policies and views of their party. Once consensus is reached between the Six Parties, the ICH EWG performs a sign off of the draft ICH guideline or recommendations with the status of ICH Step 1 for transmission to the ICH SC.

ICH STEP 2: START OF REGULATORY ACTION

The ICH SC further, discusses if there is sufficient scientific accord to concur with the draft ICH guideline or recommendations for transmission to the authorities in each of the three ICH regions. If they agree, then each ICH party performs a sign off at the level of the ICH SC, assigning the status of ICH Step 2 to the draft ICH guideline or recommendations.

ICH STEP 3: REGULATORY CONSULTATION

Pursuant to ICH Step 2, *i.e* after each party performing a sign off at the level of ICH SC, The draft ICH guideline or recommendations are then presented to the authorities in each of the three ICH regions. This is for the draft ICH guideline or recommendations for release for public consultation according to the rules established in each region for public consultation of guidance documents. Within each ICH region, comments are collected from all interested parties and discussed by the Contact Network that is mentined above. The draft ICH guideline or recommendations are also published by the ICH Secretariat for comments from authorities, industry associations and interested parties outside the ICH regions to be submitted to WHO or IFPMA. Thus the process also in this manner receives unbiased comments from all significant authorities who are connected to drug safety. Out of the three ICH Topic Leaders from the authorities, an ICH Regulatory Rapporteur is designated to draw up the final draft ICH guideline or recommendations, taking into account all comments received during the consultation, as considered relevant by the respective Contact Network. The final draft ICH guideline or recommendations are signed off by the three ICH Topic Leaders from the authorities and transmitted to the ICH SC.

ICH STEP 4: ADOPTION OF TRIPARTITE ICH GUIDELINE OR RECOMMENDATIONS

The final draft ICH guideline or recommendations and a report on the comments received during the consultation are presented by the ICH Regulatory Rapporteur to the ICH SC for consideration as to whether the consensus achieved at ICH Step 2 has been substantially altered in the final draft. If not, the ICH SC adopts the ICH guideline or recommendations with a status of ICH Step 4 for recommendation for adoption by the authorities in the three ICH regions. If yes, the ICH SC considers the alterations in the final draft, and if all parties are satisfied, adopts it with the status of ICH Step 4. If one or more parties from industry are of the opinion that the draft has been substantially altered or introduces new issues, the parties from the authorities may agree to further consultation.

ICH STEP 5: IMPLEMENTATION OF ICH GUIDELINE OR RECOMMENDATIONS

Immediately after ICH Step 4, the ICH guideline or recommendations are processed for adoption by the authorities and implementation in the three ICH regions according to the rules established in each region for any guidance documents.

A GLIMPSE AT PRE-MARKETING TRIALS

Albeit, for every new drug that enters market, there is a set procedure of clinical trials (involving four phases) being conducted, but still it does not serve as a guarantee that the drug will be safe enough to prevent any risks that a patient can suffer in real life situations during consumption of a medication.

Clinical development of medicines includes 4 phases:

1. ***Phase I:*** This includes 20–50 healthy volunteers to gather preliminary data.
2. ***Phase II:*** 150–350 patients to determine safety and dosage recommendations.
3. ***Phase III:*** 250–4000 more varied patient groups to determine the short term safety and efficacy.
4. ***Phase IV:*** Post approval studies to determine specific safety issues.

Drug safety monitoring in clinical trials ensures the safety of the participants and a constant assessment of the risks and the benefits associated with Investigational product. Investigational medicinal products basically includes either unauthorized products still under investigation or authorized products under investigation for new indications or in dosages other than those recommended by the product information. Pharmacovigilance with regards to clinical trials phase I to III covers drug safety monitoring and evaluation of all adverse events with or without a causal relationship to the investigational medicinal product and any adverse drug reaction to concomitant medication. In oncology clinical trials which involves the patients with unfavourable prognosis, where emphasis is placed on survival, a risk benefit ratio assessment is very important. Specifically taking into consideration, the advancements in research for more effective chemotherapeutics, which comprises a wide spectrum of new approaches, is slow and the benefits of new treatments over less toxic standard approaches have been modest. The question that needs to be addressed in such a scenario is whether or not the small improvements in overall survival compensate for the additional discomfort experienced by the patient.

Throughout Europe, the adverse event documentation and reporting in clinical trials has been harmonized by implementation of the Clinical Directive 2001/20/EC into national law, which is mentioned in Table 3 below. Reporting Serious Unexpected Suspected Adverse Reactions (SUSARS) clinical trials to competent authorities and ethics committees is made time bound and has been enforced (no later than 7 days for deaths and life-threatening adverse reactions and 15 days for all others). The objective is thus to identify and concentrate on SUSAR, allowing for annual review and revision (Directive 2001/28/EC) of the product information (Investigator Brochure or Summary of Product Characteristics (SmPC) by the pharmaceutical industry (MAH). In addition adverse drug reactions associated with concomitant medication administered in clinical trials, where the sponsor is not the marketing authorization holder, should be reported either directly to competent authorities or to the marketing authorization holder of the concomitant medication so as regulatory requirements can be met and the serious adverse drug reactions can be reported to the competent authorities within 15 days.

Table 3: The clinical trials safety regulations

Regulations for safety monitoring in clinical trials
Directive 2001/20/EC Directive 2001/20/EG of the European Parliament and of the Council on the approximation of the laws, regulations and administrative provisions of the Member States relating to implementation of good clinical practice in the conduct of clinical trials on medicinal products for human use. Official Journal of the European Communities' (L121, pp34-44).
ENTR/CT 3 Brussels April 2004 Detailed guidance on the collection, verification and presentation of adverse reaction reports arising from clinical trials on medicinal products for human use. A guidance written in request of Article 18 of Directive 2001/20/EC
ENTR/CT 4 Brussels April 2004 EudraVigilance Clinical Trial Module - Detailed guidance on the European Database of Suspected Unexpected Serious Adverse Reactions. A guidance written in request of Article 17.3(a) of Directive 2001/20/EC
ENTR/CT 5 Brussels April 2004 Detailed Guidance on the European Clinical Trials Database (EudraCTDatabase). A guidance written in request of Article 11 of the Directive 2001/20/EC
E6 CPMP/ICH/135/95 ICH Topic E6 Guideline for Good Clinical Practice and CPMP/ICH/135/95 Note for Guidance on Good Clinical Practice
E2A CPMP/ICH/377/95 Clinical Safety Data Management: Definitions and Standards for Expedited Reporting
E2BM CPMP/ICH/287/95 Data Elements for Transmission of Individual Case Safety Reports (ICSR) (2002). E2B (M) Data Elements for Transmission of ICSR (2004 Q & A)
E2B/M2 CPMP/ICH/285/95 Maintenance of the Clinical Safety Data Management including the Maintenance of the Electronic Transmission of ICSR Message Specification
CIOMS Working Group V Current Challenges in Pharmacovigilance: Pragmatic Approaches
CIOMS Working Group VI Management of Safety Information from Clinical Trials

Once onto the market, the product leaves the secure and protected scientific ambience of clinical trials and is legally set free for the consumption by the general population. Until then, the product was put to test on few subjects for assessing the short term safety and efficacy. Hence it is essential that new and medically still evolving treatments are monitored for their effectiveness and safety in real life conditions post release. Adverse effects, interactions with food and other medicines and allied risk factors come to light during the years after release of the medicine. More information is generally needed with regard to special population groups, *viz:* children, pregnant women and elderly and about the safety and efficacy of chronic use, especially in combination with other medicines. Thus after registration of the product and once it is onto the market, the Phase IV post approval and spontaneous reporting is conducted to tackle the safety concerns. The decision to approve a drug is based on its benefit-risk balance within the conditions specified in the product labeling which is in accordance to the information available at the time of approval. Thus, risk assessment during product development should be conducted in a thorough and rigorous manner; however, it is impossible to identify all safety concerns during clinical trials. Once a product is marketed, there is generally a large increase in the number of patients exposed in a shorter time frame, including those with co-morbid conditions and those being treated with concomitant medical products. The information related to safety profile of the product can vary over time, like in case of early postmarketing period the product might be used in settings different from clinical trials. Consequently, postmarketing safety data collection and risk assessment based on observational data are vital for evaluating and characterizing a product's risk profile and for making informed decisions on risk minimization. The new information that is generated, once the product is marketed can have an impact on the benefits or risks of the product. This benefit-risk balance can be improved by reducing risks to patients through effective pharmacovigilance. Thus in a timely manner, information feedback can be provided to the users.

DRUG SAFETY

For the pharmaceutical industry, pharmacovigilance is the post-marketing surveillance of the safety of authorized commercialised medicinal products during their life on the market. It includes safety monitoring and evaluation of suspected adverse drug reactions from phase IV clinical trials, observational non-interventional studies *e.g.* postmarketing surveillance studies, pharmacoepidemiologic studies, solicited reports from surveys, registries, patient diaries etc., literature sources and spontaneous reports from healthcare professionals and includes assessment of quality complaints. The European Pharmacovigilance Guidelines regulate the responsibilities of the pharmaceutical industry to establish a reliable pharmacovigilance system with continual monitoring of drug safety (including regular literature database searches of *e.g.* Medline, Embase), prompt reporting to the competent authorities (within 15 days of receipt of information), detection of signals with a timely initiation of a risk management plan. The pharmacovigilance guideline requires a named "qualified person" with medical qualification or direct access to medical expertise to organise and coordinate safety procedures and risk management including drug recall within the pharmaceutical firm. Inspections will be initiated by the European Medicines Evaluation Agency (EMEA) to check compliance of the pharmaceutical industry with the pharmacovigilance guidelines and with the authority to release warnings, public notices of the offence including the name of the Marketing Authorisation Holder and if appropriate take legal action (penal offence and fines). Competent authorities must co-operate and exchange information with one another. This has been facilitated by the establishment of the EMEA Eudravigilance Database and provision for electronic transfer of data. This is a central computer database established by the EMEA in December 2001, in London, which contains adverse reaction reports to medicines licensed across Europe. Competent authorities, EMEA and European Commission have access to this database. In addition the Marketing Authorisation Holder is legally bound at regular intervals following the licensing of the product to prepare a Periodic Safety Update Report on the licensing status of the product in the global market, detailed information on drug safety with a systematic analysis and evaluation of the risk benefit profile based on cumulative data from all sources, including national and international publications as well as a report on any necessary consequences.

Pharmacovigilance is defined as the science and activities relating to the detection, assessment, understanding and prevention of adverse effects or any other drug related problems. PV studies the long term and short term adverse drug reaction or simply stated side effects of medicines. PV system involves collection, monitoring, researching upon, assessing and evaluating information received from health care practitioners, such as doctors, pharmacists, nurses and other health care professionals for understanding the ADR. PV definition includes monitoring of all pharmaceutical drugs and also other medical products including vaccines, X-ray contrast media, traditional and herbal medicines etc, especially when the reaction is unusual, potentially serious or clinically significant.

Objectives of Pharmacovigilance are enlisted below:

- To improve patient care, public health and safety in relation to the use of medicines and all medical and paramedical interventions.
- To evaluate benefit, harm, effectiveness and risk of medicines.
- To encourage the safe, rational and more effective use of medicines.
- To promote understanding, education and clinical training in pharmacovigilance and its effective communication to public.

Pharmacovigilance is mainly governed by

- The pharmaceutical industry (prime responsibility)
- Competent (regulatory) authorities (http://heads.medagencies.org/)
- WHO collaborating Centre for International Drug Monitoring (in Uppsala)
- Council for International Organization of Medical Sciences - CIOMS Working Groups on drug safety play an advisory role in harmonization of pharmacovigilance practices.

Since the essence of Pharmacovigilance is to assess the benefit-risk ratio and thereby help patients receive a more effective and safe care in terms of the therapy given to them, PV is now spreading wings into the alternative system of medicine as well. This is because adverse effects related to a particular therapy type may be a possibility irrespective of the kind of medicines used. Thus herbal, traditional and complementary medicines, blood products, biologicals, medical devices and vaccines have been recent inclusions into the pharmacovigilance purview. Herbal and traditional medicine needs incorporation within a regulatory framework. Safety concerns are associated with such medicines but the general myth quotes natural means safe. But there are examples of traditional and herbal medicines being adulterated or contaminated with allopathic medicines, chemicals such as corticosteroids, non steroidal anti-inflammatory agents and heavy metals. Self medication aggravates the risk to patients and when they are used in conjunction with other medicines there is the potential of serious adverse drug interactions. Thus there is a need for these medicines to be governed by standards of safety, quality and efficacy on par with other pharmaceutical products.

Thus, there needs to be regulations in place so that drug safety issues are handled more efficiently and adequately. There is an ever increasing regulatory activity in the field of drug safety and risk management, but three key issues dominate the discussion on drug safety, they being:

- Risk management plans
- Safety surveillance and signal detection
- Establishment and continuous monitoring of benefit-risk relationship

Safety and risk management systems need to be strategically integrated alongside business processes. Approach which not only delivers but also controls the overall risk management should be existent with all companies including specifically small and midsize startup companies. Absence of such a form can stall the success of development pipelines and business models. This is because a single drug withdrawal from the market due to safety issues can be really costly for a company in terms of returns.

Portfolio's Success

From the perspective of R & D companies, the stake holders can be broadly categorized into two, *viz*: internal and external. Internal include all elements which are affected by the success or nonsuccess of R & D activities, they being clinical department, drug safety, regulatory, medical, finance, legal, human resources, sales plus marketing and global financial community or investors. The external stakeholders comprise patients and healthcare providers, regulatory and government agencies, professional organizations, policy makers, legal firms, pharmacies and other drug retailers. And all of them for differing reasons have an interest for the investigational product. The internal misalignment between different functions within the company is matched by a perceived or actual conflict of interest between the pharmaceutical industry, regulatory bodies, patient groups and health professionals. This in turn has developed into a major problem for pharmaco-vigilance and return on investment. Government and public don't believe pharmaceutical and biotechnology companies to get risk management right. Internal competition and disconnect has led to an external loss of credibility. And in the process, the perception that biopharmaceutical companies is trying to hide information on product risk gets confirmed. But ultimately, one thing needs to be realized that the health care sector is directly linked to consumer satisfaction. And hence if consumers *i.e* patients suffer adversely due to the risk of a product outweighing the benefit aspect then this results in failure of the product in market. Further the consumer starts getting skeptical of the health care sector of a country.

Thus the following measures needs to be adopted by the companies involved in researching and manufacturing of a healthcare product:

- Safety and risk management strategy and infrastructure for risk limitation.
- Clinical development operations integrated with the pharmaco-vigilance value chain.
- Integration of risk communication with public risk perception for risk management.

Again it is not necessary that the safety issues that arise because of a product *i.e* an adverse reaction due to the drug is solely because of the drug in question. It might be due to many factors, including usage, administration error, patient related errors etc. Thus, some special cases are also considered while data processing of the safety issues such as:

- Lack of efficacy reports
- Medication error reports
- Accidental administration
- Substandard medicines
- Use of medicines for indications that are not approved and for which there are inadequate scientific basis.
- Acute and chronic poisoning cases
- Assessment of drug related mortality
- Abuse and misuse of medicines

- Adverse interactions of medicines with chemicals, other medicines and food.

There are regional variation in the occurrences of Adverse Drug Reactions (ADRs) and other drug related problems. These disparities may be attributed to the differences in diseases and prescribing practices, genetics, diet, traditions of the people, drug manufacturing processes used which in turn influence the product quality and composition, drug distribution and use including indications, dose and availability. Additionally, there has been a growing awareness of extending the scope of pharmacovigilance beyond the strict confines of detecting new signals of safety concerns. Globalization, consumerism, explosion in free trade and communication across borders and increasing use of internet have given rise to new safety issues such as:

- Increasing self medication practices
- Illegal sale of medicines and drugs of abuse over internet.
- Unsafe drug donation practices
- Manufacture and sale of counterfeit and substandard medicines
- Increasing use of traditional medicines and herbal medicines with other medicines with possibility of adverse reactions.

PV in Europe is coordinated by the European Medicines Agency (EMA) and conducted by the National Competent Authorities (NCAs). The database comprising all suspected serious adverse drug reactions observed in European region is maintained and developed by the EMA. In United States, there are three branches of the pharmacovigilance system, *i.e* FDA, the pharmaceutical manufacturers and the academic non profit organizations like RADAR and public citizen. The USFDA receives reports about ADRs and takes appropriate actions for drug safety. In India the main governing authority is the Central Drugs Standard Control Organization (CDSCO), Ministry of health and family welfare, which forms the top of the pharmacovigilance structure. Under this there are two zonal pharmacovigilance centers, *i.e* Seth GS medical college, Mumbai and AIIMS, New Delhi.

Few developing countries, however, have the structures, systems, or resources in place to support medicine safety activities, and countries often lack unbiased, evidence-based information to help guide treatment decisions and promote rational—that is, safe, effective, and cost-effective—use of medicines. In addition, sustained budgetary support for pharmacovigilance and medicine safety activities is generally lacking. With augmented access to vital medicines comes a greater need to monitor and promote the safety and effectiveness of these medicines.

2

Methods in Pharmacovigilance

As we have seen in the previous chapter, pharmacovigilance is all about studying the safety issues pertaining to a particular drug whilst it is used by public in a real life situation. The intrinsic properties of the drug rather than the way in which it is used and the rarity with which a drug gives rise to an adverse reaction has led to a lot of thought provoking discussions by regulators, pharmaceutical companies, pharmacovigilators to arrive at fool proof processes and concrete steps that may lead to recognizing safety signals in the very beginning of the drug development process and thereby minimizing risks.

There have been instances where despite of a lot of efforts from the phamaceutical companies, there have been reported adverse reactions with regards to a product. Like for instance, the reported associations between MMR vaccines, inflammatory bowel disease and autism have caused great concerns about all vaccines in parents.

But one thing that needs to be borne in mind is while we expect a higher benefit: risk ratio, anticipating zero risks out of a drug and that too a new drug, molecule is rather unrealistic. It should always be remembered that only a few hundreds to thousands of the population for a given therapeutic category have been exposed to the new drug before the product is marketed. The emergence of various systems in pharmacovigilance, the hard work and initiatives taken by CIOMS, the various methods of drug safety reporting are all various ventures into making the pharmacovigilance system robust and safe ensuring a patient "a good nights sleep".

Thus we shall in this chapter probe into the various methods of pharmacovigilance coined till date. Pharmacovigilance methods are classified based on the sources from where the adverse events are reported. Dependent on if the information is received from unsolicited communication by health care professionals or consumers, online reporting of adverse events, data from specific patient subgroups, observational studies etc, the pharmacovigilance methods are classified into various types.

The adverse event reports can be obtained from various sources and can be categorized into different methods. The various pharmacovigilance methods include:

- Passive surveillance
- Stimulated reporting
- Active surveillance
- Comparative observational studies
- Targeted clinical investigations
- Descriptive studies

Thus the reports received from these sources give a detailed narration about the safety issues pertaining to a patient. A case report is complete data on an adverse event. An assessment of the safety issue with regard to a drug is done by analyzing the case report. Thus, FDA recommends that sponsors make reasonable attempt to obtain complete information for case assessment initially or subsequent follow up in case of serious events.

A complete case report must include details about Patient, Adverse event, Drug exposure and Source. The basic components of a case report are:

- ***Patient:*** Patient characteristics comprises demographic information (Age, sex, race), baseline medical condition prior to product therapy, co-morbid conditions, use of concomitant medications, relevant family medical history of diseases and presence of other risk factors.

- ***Adverse event:*** Description of adverse event includes aspect, place, severity and diagnosis including time to onset of signs or symptoms, outcome, course, time relationship: re-challenge and de-challenge, Laboratory data with respect to the event.
- ***Drug exposure (suspected and other):*** Suspected and concomitant product therapy details (*i.e.*, dose, indication, generic ingredients, batch number, lot number, schedule, dates which include duration and interval), including over-the-counter medications, dietary supplements, and recently discontinued medications forms the information related to Drug exposure.
- ***Source:*** Source is necessary to understand that who supplied the details regarding the adverse event/ adverse reaction.

As seen above Patient Demographics, Adverse event information, Drug exposure details, and source of the report form the pillars to make a case report complete. However there are some more details which the case report should ideally include. Thus case reports should also include the following elements, apart from the above mentioned components:

1. Documentation of the diagnosis of the events, including methods used to make the diagnosis;
2. Clinical course of the event and patient outcomes (*e.g.*, hospitalization or death)
3. Relevant therapeutic measures and laboratory data at baseline, during therapy, and subsequent to therapy, including blood levels, as appropriate;
4. Information about response to de-challenge and re-challenge; and
5. Any other relevant information (*e.g.*, other details relating to the event or information on benefits received by the patient, if important to the assessment of the event).

The above information gives data about the other events along with the main event that has occurred if any. Also the diagnostic method provides facts about the accuracy of the information as well. The seriousness and fatality of the event is understood by the information such as hospitalization and/or death. Response to de-challenge and re-challenge provides information regarding the relationship of the drug to the event that has occurred. In Re-challenge, the assessment of the patient's condition is done with respect to continuation of drug in question to the patient and de-challenge is the effect of discontinuation of the drug to the patient. Additional lab details including blood levels, hemoglobin content, RBC value, WBC count etc provides information regarding meticulous details on condition of the patient. Thus in other words this listed information helps in the holistic assessment of the adverse event that has transpired.

The various pharmacovigilance methods are enlisted below:

- Passive surveillance
- Stimulated reporting
- Active surveillance
- Comparative observational studies
- Targeted clinical investigations
- Descriptive studies

These methods are discussed elaborately further in the chapter:

Hypothesis generating methods: Is inclusive of Spontaneous reporting, Prescription event monitoring methods.

Hypothesis testing methods: Is inclusive of Case control & Crossover, Cohort, Randomized Clinical methods.

1. ***Passive surveillance:*** Spontaneous reports and case series form part of the passive surveillance method.

   A. *Spontaneous reporting:* This is a structured system for reporting of suspected adverse reactions. The report is an unsolicited communication by health care professionals or consumers to a company, regulatory authority or other organization. This is not derived from a study or any organized data collection scheme. It is a case report which is a notification from the practitioner regarding a patient with a disorder that is suspected to be drug related. Medical secrecy and privacy is maintained in such type of reporting. Spontaneous reports can also provide important information pertaining to at risk groups, risk factors, clinical features of known serious adverse drug reactions. There are many methods for detecting signals from spontaneous reports which include proportional reporting ratio, Bayesian technique, data mining. These have been discussed in detail in the next chapter.

Spontaneous reporting being an unsolicited communication operates for all drugs throughout their lifetime and is the only affordable method of detecting really rare ADRs. Since the data reported from a spontaneous reporting system deals with a real life case or real life patient, even the suspicions are not ignored and are given due consideration. Thus all reports are treated as hypothesis. The reporter base ecompasses a wide range, viz: nurses, pharmacists, other health care professionals and patients. This reporting system is invaluable because it has led to the identification and verification of many unexpected serious ADRs and it is essential that health professionals should be provided with the means of reporting their suspicions. Careful analysis of all reported suspected reactions to a particular drug may direct the suspectedness to a particular pool or population of people.

The main lacuna with this method is that there is under-reporting, and the data provide a 'numerator' (the number of reports of each suspected reaction) only. These findings have resulted in many marketed drugs being withdrawn or additional information being provided to guide safer use of the product.

Some of the advantages of spontaneous reporting are listed below:

- Effective and cheap method
- Wide coverage by considering all patients, all drugs and all adverse reactions
- Continuous and rapid.

Limitations of spontaneous reporting include:

- Under-reporting and bias
- Drug consumption data being available is questionable
- No quantitative assessment
- Comparison of drugs is difficult
- No proof of causality exists
- Often further study is needed like hypothesis testing and evaluation

Certain elements which need to be considered while reporting are:

- Unknown and unexpected reactions must be reported.
- Reactions with respect to new drugs must be reported promptly.
- Serious reactions even when they are known, like Fatal & life threatening, hospitalization, persistent incapacity or disability, dependence and malformations must be reported immediately.
- Unexpected beneficial effects and ineffectiveness must also be reported.

Data assessment of information in hand is done by individual case report assessment and aggregated reports assessment coupled with interpretation. Individual case report assessment must include the relevance of report, coding, quality of documentation, case follow-up and case causality assessment. The aggregated report interpretation must comprise of signal detection, studying interactions and risk factors, serial clinico-pathological study and frequency estimation. Case follow-ups are essential to provide missing data in previous reports, additional laboratory data and pathology records, outcome data in case the patient was not recovered when initial case was reported, underlying disease condition if any and verification of findings.

The central authority can be notified about the suspected ADRs that are detected by Physicians, other health care professionals or patients. Since 1964, the "yellow card" has been used in the United Kingdom for the purpose of reporting. FP10 prescriptions pads, the British National Formulary and other sources are other means of reporting. The MedWatch form in United States are made available to health professionals for reporting.

A variety of formal epidemiological studies can be undertaken to generate or test hypotheses.

B. *Case series:* Evidence of an association between a drug and an adverse event is provided by case series of reports. These are generally spontaneously reported distinct adverse events which are more associated with the drug therapy like, anaphylaxis, aplastic anemia, toxic epidermal necrolysis and Steven Johnson syndrome. There needs to be a detailed and rapid follow up done by sponsors when such events are spontaneously reported.

2. ***Stimulated reporting:*** This method includes online reporting of adverse events based on pre-designed method for new products or for limited time periods. This type of reporting in the early marketing phase can enable companies to notify healthcare professionals of new therapies and provide safety information early in use by the general population. In this case accurate incidence rates are not generated but reporting rates can be estimated. Certain limitations of such a method are selective reporting and incomplete information.
3. ***Active surveillance:*** This method includes a pre-organized process to establish completely the number of adverse events. In this case report is obtained from various means like:

   A. *Sentinel sites:* Here the data from specific patient subgroups, drug abuse information can be procured. Selection bias, small number of patients and increased costs are some of the limitations of this type. Risks associated with orphan drug consumption can be identified by intensive monitoring of sentinel sites.

   B. *Drug event monitoring:* Here a questionnaire is sent to prescribing physician or patients who are identified by either electronic prescription data or automated health insurance claims. The questionnaire generally contains information on patient demographics, indication for treatment and duration of therapy, dosage, clinical events and reasons for discontinuation. Important signals can be obscured by poor response rates and unfocused nature of data collection.

   C. *Registries:* List of patients with similar set of characteristics is called a registry. They could be disease registry where the characteristic is same disease or drug registry where the patients are exposed to a specific drug. In disease registries for instance, a particular disorder wich is drug induced is taken into consideration. Chloramphenicol related aplastic anaemia and stilboestrol related vaginal adenocarcinoma are initiatives related to disease registries.

4. ***Comparative observational studies:*** Observational study designs are useful in validating signals from spontaneous reports or case series. Cross sectional studies, case control studies and cohort studies (retrospective and prospective) are some of the types of comparative observational designs.

   A. *Cross sectional study:* This type of study involves data collection on a population of patients at a single point in time regardless of exposure or disease status. Prevalence of a disease at one time point, trends over time can be examined in this case but relationship between drug exposure and outcome cannot be directly established.

   B. *Case control study:* Herein, cases of disease or events are identified and controls without the disease or events are selected from source population that give rise to cases. The controls are selected in such a way that the prevalence of exposure among the controls represents the prevalence of exposure in the source population. Odds ratio is used to compare the exposure status of the two groups which gives an estimate of the relative risk of disease in two groups. These studies give an insight into the association between drug and one specific rare adverse event and alongside gives information about the risk factors for adverse events.

   C. *Cohort study:* In this type of study, population at risk for the disease or event is followed over time for the occurrence of the same. During this follow up, the patient might be exposed at one time point and may be unexposed at the other time point. Incidence rates can be evaluated since the population exposure is known.

5. ***Targeted clinical investigations:*** Mechanism of action for adverse reaction is assessed in cases wherein there is significant risk identified from pre-approval clinical trials. Further clinical studies are carried out or in some instances also pharmacokinetic and pharmacodynamic studies may be performed to examine if the specific dosage regimen/dose can put patients at increased risk of adverse events. Potential drug-drug interactions and food-drug interactions can be investigated form pharmacological properties and the expected use of drug in general practice.

6. ***Descriptive studies:*** Background rate of outcome events and establishing prevalence of the use of drugs in specified populations are done in this study. This could be performed by using natural history of disease or drug utilization study.

The reports obtained from various sources are stored accordingly in appropriate databases which are as listed below:

1. ***Spontaneous reporting databases:*** Involuntary reporting of a possible adverse drug reaction by healthcare providers to governmental agencies or drug companies is spontaneous reporting. This passive system has unpredictable reporting as a limitation, with more frequent reporting for unusual reactions, reactions for new drugs and serious reactions. Furthermore, the accuracy of the data contained within the reports is uncertain. However, spontaneous reporting databases do contain large amounts of data; these databases can therefore be mined to obtain details of adverse drug events.
2. ***Prescription event monitoring databases:*** This Prescription event monitoring combines the features of spontaneous reporting and public health surveillance with aspects of formal epidemiological studies. Within the British National Health Service (NHS), prescriptions written by physicians are sent to a central Prescription Pricing Authority (PPA) after dispensing. This is particularly followed in United Kingdom (UK) and New Zealand. PEM in the United Kingdom and a similar programme in New Zealand are unique in providing a monitored-release programme that can detect or help refute new signals in the early life of a medicine. In the UK, Prescription Event monitoring system takes advantage of the aspects of the British National Health Service (NHS). The PPA then forwards the confidential copies of certain prescriptions for newly introduced monitored drugs to the Drug Safety Research Unit (DSRU). A green form questionnaire is then sent by the DSRU to the General Practitioner (GP) who wrote the original prescription. This is sent six or twelve months after the first prescription is given for an individual drug to an individual patient. Thus, the whole idea of PEM is to provide for 'exposure data' showing which patients have been exposed to the drug being monitored. Followed by the green forms giving information about the 'outcome data' showing any events noted during the period of

monitoring. Also special cases such as events in pregnant women, deaths or other significant events can be followed up by contact between the DSRU and the prescribing doctor who holds, within the NHS, the lifetime medical record of all of his or her registered patients. Also the data interpretation is neither difficult nor biased because the physicians decision regarding prescription to individual patients are not interfered. Both the numerator (the number of reports) and a denominator (the number of patients exposed), that are collected over a precisely known period of observation can be obtained from such a system of Prescription Event Monitoring. But statistically only 50–70% of the green forms are returned, and the experience of the patients whose forms are not returned may differ from those returned. Also, PEM limits follow-up to 6 or 12 months and hence it cannot identify events of long latency. Again this method does not help investigate the genetic and metabolic features of those patients who produce these very rare type B adverse reactions. Thus the inborn errors of metabolism or other rarities present in a given patient that reflects features of the patient rather than the drug may not be confirmed. But the physicians must continue to support the scheme by returning those green forms that they receive for effective functioning of PEM and detecting early ADRS.

Select group of patients are exposed to a specific drug, which may also be a new drug for a limited period of time. High quality data is thereby collected and stored in Prescription event monitoring (PEM) databases. The adverse event information is provided by family doctors in this case. A limitation of PEM database mining is the lack of an adequate control group, as the database contains details of clusters of patients exposed to certain drugs.

3. ***Linked administrative databases:*** The record is available at a relatively small additional cost and is not subject to recall or interviewer bias. The completeness of details in this case, such as diagnoses, is questionable in many circumstances, and the data tends to apply only to elderly or low-income populations and so may not be representative of the whole population. Medicaid in the U.S is an example of Large linked health administrative databases that contain data on millions of subjects and may also be used as a source for data mining.

4. ***Electronic medical records:*** Utilization of tobacco products, smoking and nonprescription drugs, symptoms and signs, laboratory data and social circumstances are present in the Electronic medical records (EMR). This encompasses a smaller number of patients. Because of the large number and detail of the variables, which can be combined to generate new diagnoses or adverse events, hypotheses can be explored that are not restricted to existing diagnoses.
5. ***Other databases:*** Clinical trials databases and specialist databases, such as overdose or toxicology databases, may also contain valuable information. Data retrieved from databases needs to undergo data preprocessing, which involves data sampling and data quality verification to ensure it is clean and well described. Medical data can contain erroneous data, such as ages of 120 years rather than 20 years or a documentation of hysterectomy in males. New variables of interest to be used in the analysis can be generated from the data.

As we have seen that pharmacovigilance has steadily progressed in the due course of around five and a half decades from the nascent stage it was at the time of thalidomide disaster. With evolution came in many more methods of reporting adverse reactions. Albeit, these methods have their own limitations, but they are definitely going to be overcome with more awareness of drug safety amongst all stake holders with regards drug safety.

3

Adverse Drug Reactions

Adverse drug reactions (ADRs) are among the leading causes of mortality. Apart from the inherent risk associated with products themselves, individual patients may exhibit specific and unpredictable sensitivities to a given medication. Information about rare but serious adverse reactions, chronic toxicity, use in special groups (such as children, the elderly or pregnant women) is often incomplete or unavailable. Moreover, if more than one medicine is prescribed, there is a risk of drug-drug interaction. Thus considerable skill is required from the practitioner to prescribe the best and safest medicine for a given individual. Mechanisms for evaluating and monitoring the safety of medicines in clinical use are vital for improving public health. This can be accomplished by having a well structured and systematic pharmacovigilance system.

Adverse drug reaction is defined as an appreciably harmful or unpleasant interaction resulting from an intervention related to the use of a medicinal product, which foretells hazard from future administration and warrants prevention or specific treatment or alteration of the dosage regimen or withdrawal of the product. Whereas an adverse event refers to an untoward effect following drug exposure but not necessarily caused by the medicine. By the time the drug is marketed only a handful of 1500 to 3000 patients are exposed to the drug and resulting in only those adverse reactions occuring at a frequency of greater than 1 in 500–1000 being reported at the time of licensing.

ADR means a response which is noxious and unintended and which occurs at doses normally used in humans for the prophylaxis, diagnosis or therapy of disease or for the modification of physiological function. A reaction, contrary to an event is characterized by the fact that a causal relationship between the drug and the occurrence is suspected, *i.e.* judged possible by the reporting or reviewing healthcare professional. Adverse event is any untoward medical occurrence that may be present during the treatment with a pharmaceutical product but which does not necessarily have a causal relationship with this treatment.

Adverse reactions is often viewed, incorrectly, as 'side effects' and thus as distractions from patients' and doctors' priorities. Learning about the scope and severity of ADRs should start early in professional training. Good safety monitoring enables healthcare practitioners to take fuller responsibility for the medicines they use. It improves clinical efficacy and the confidence with which they and their patients use medicines. Focus needs to be given to training health professionals in diagnosis, management and prevention of ADRs. Identification of less obvious adverse effects requires clinical alertness, accurate diagnosis and an understanding of the principles of causality assessment. Health professionals are more likely to identify and report important ADRs if they can diagnose, manage and prevent such reactions.

Adverse drug reactions which are unwanted effects of medicines have significant consequences for the individual and have a major impact on public health. Thus adverse reactions to medicines contribute majorly to serious illness and early death. There are instances wherein the adverse effects are unavoidable or unpredictable, but with a correct approach to using medicines, the occurence of adverse drug reactions can be reduced considerably. As discussed earlier, adverse drug reactions and adverse events are two different terms and are not interchangeable. Adverse drug reaction can be attributed as a reaction to a particular drug, whereas an adverse event simply describes an unwanted outcome that occurs, regardless of whether a medicine has been used or is implicated.

Clinical trials involve a few thousand patients at most and based on the results from these clinical trials licenses are granted for marketing them. The limitation associated with such trials are that all the adverse events may not happen in the limited set of patients recruited for the trials and all the more the rarer ones remain undisclosed. The screened patients therefore may not reflect real life situations exposed to a given new drug molecule. The long-term adverse effects are not revealed in Clinical trials. Thus continuous monitoring of marketed drug which is given to many patients in real life situations may bring into picture an adverse event/s that has resulted from a particular drug. This may also reveal at many occassions rare adverse effects which are serious enough to warrant additional precautions or even withdrawal of a medicine from the market.

Enrolment methods and exclusion criteria for clinical trials can result in under-representation of some sections of patient population. The trial findings may therefore have limited applicability to many patients seen in clinical practice. Despite efforts to improve population representation in trials, groups that may be poorly represented include:

- those at extremes of age: paediatric and elderly patients
- women, especially pregnant or breast-feeding women who are generally excluded
- patients with one or more co-morbid conditions (and who are using other medicines concomitantly); those with significant renal or hepatic impairment are often under-represented
- patients from ethnic minorities.

Thus the limitations that clinical trials provide whilst identifying adverse events are:

- Limited exposure of patients to the new drug molecule
- Lack of real life situation
- Adverse events/rare adverse events which may get revealed only after prolonged exposure.
- The medical history of patients which are individualistic in nature
- Concomitant medications which are administered along with the suspect drug. This may vary from patient to patient under real life situations.
- Under-representation of particular pool of patients due to exclusion criteria and enrolment methods.

Complete active participation of health professionals is necessary in further strengthening the pharmacovigilance system, thus ensuring that medicines are selected and used in its full positive capacity. The harm that might precipitate due to adverse reactions must be considered meticulously and analyzed thoroughly. An untoward event detected as a suspected adverse effect to one or more medicines must be promptly reported. Reporting such effects can allow pharmacovigilance centres to fully assess the significance of the effect and to act on the findings. The health care professionals can help in further mitigation of harm either through spontaneous adverse-effect reporting systems or by participating in active surveillance schemes.

Risk management is one important aspect of a structured pharmacovigilance system needs to be carefully handled by pharmaceutical companies so that due responsibility is taken for identifying risk with their products and for taking necessary actions to mitigate the risk. PSURs are one such approach to send across reports of adverse reactions to appropriate medicines regulators. This section will be dealt with in detail in subsequent chapters.

Medicines and Healthcare products Regulatory Agency (MHRA) and the European Medicines Agency are the medicine regulators of UK and they play a major role for pharmacovigilance in the UK.

The MHRA operates in the following manner:

- The Yellow Card Scheme for collecting spontaneous reports of adverse effects
- Monitors clinical literature for information on potential harm from medicines
- Assesses reports of suspected adverse effects
- Uses its regulatory powers to ensure that marketing authorisations reflect current knowledge on potential harm
- Communicates new information on risks and their management.

The **Summary of Product Characteristics (SmPC, SPC)**, which is issued for each licensed medicine, lists adverse effects of the medicine in the context of other prescribing information such as indications, dose, contraindications, warnings, and interactions. Adverse effects are included on the basis of evidence from initial clinical trials. New informaton that emerges from post marketing (post authorisation) studies and from adverse effects are accordingly updated in the Adverse effect list and thus the list is regularly updated.

In SmPCs, adverse effects are generally grouped by body systems and are shown with the frequency parameters like very common, common, uncommon, rare and very rare. Further the percentages of their occurrence are added along with respective parameters, *viz*:

Very common (> 10%), Common (1–10%),
Uncommon (0.1–1%), Rare (0.01–0.1%), and
Very rare (< 0.01%).

The following elements are likely to reduce significantly the risks of adverse effects and their severity:

- An adequate drug history of the patient
- Rational prescribing and dispensing
- Proper counselling
- The provision of clear and understandable drug information.

The British National Formulary (BNF) which provides information on medicines, including their adverse effects ('side-effects' in the BNF) are used by clinicians. It includes most of its information that is taken from SmPCs, which is also inclusive of information from other sources. Some of the very rare adverse effects are omitted. For many drug classes, the BNF groups adverse effects that apply to the class as a whole. A brief list of adverse effects is also provided in **MIMS** (Monthly Index of Medical Specialties).

- ***Clinical software*** used in hospitals and general practices may also include information on warnings, interactions and adverse effects of medicines. However, it is important to establish the provenence of this information and to determine how often it is updated.
- ***Patient information leaflets***, supplied with medicines and also available online, are a plain-language reflection of SmPCs and can be valuable for discussion with patients.

Reporting of an adverse event by health care professionals is a valuable step towards bettering the health care system and thus proving to be a boon to mankind which can save lives of many patients.

ADR reporting should be a must rule followed by every country worldwide. It is significant because:

- Tests in animals are insufficient to predict human safety
- Patients used in clinical trials are selected and limited in number, the conditions of use differ from those in clinical practice and the duration of use is limited.
- By the time of licensing, exposure of less than 5000 subjects to a drug allows only the more common ADR to be detected.

A larger population thus needs to be considered, so as to ensure that 1 ADR which has an incidence of 1 in 10,000 exposed individuals doesn't go unnoticed. ADR report must necessarily contain a set of four minimum information:

- An identifiable source
- A patient
- A suspected product
- A suspected reaction

BELOW MENTIONED IS A LIST OF SOME IMPORTANT DEFINITIONS

Serious Adverse Drug Reaction

A serious adverse reaction means an adverse reaction which results in death, is life threatening, requires inpatient hospitalization or prolongation of existing hospitalization, results in persistent or significant disability/incapacity or is a congenital anomaly/birth defect.

Side effect is defined as; any unintended effect of a pharmaceutical product occurring at a normal dosage which is related to the pharmacological properties of the drug.

Unexpected adverse reaction is an adverse reaction, the nature or severity of which is not consistent with domestic labeling or market authorization or expected from characteristics of the drug.

Signal may be defined as, a reported information on a possible causal relationship between adverse event and a drug, this link being unknown or incompletely documented previously. Usually more than a single report is required to generate a signal, depending on the seriousness of the event and quality of information. The publication of a signal generally implies the need for some kind of review or action.

Serious Unexpected Adverse Drug Reaction (SUADR)

Serious unexpected adverse drug reaction (SUADR) is the reaction not identified in nature, severity or frequency by the risk information provided in the clinical investigator's brochure (CIB) or on the drug label. A list of serious and unexpected reactions are stated in Table 1 below.

Table 1: Model examples of serious and unexpected adverse reactions

Medicine	*Adverse reactions*
Chloramphenicol	Aplastic anaemia
Clioquinol	Myelooptic neuropathy
Erythromycin estolate	Cholestatic hepatitis
Fluthane	Hepatocellular hepatitis
Methyldopa	Haemolytic anaemia
Oral contraceptives	Thromboembolism
Aminophenazone	Agranulocytosis
Practolol	Peritonitis
Reserpine	Depression
Statins	Rhabdomyolysis
Thalidomide	Congenital malformations

Adverse events suspected to have been caused by new drugs and drugs of current interest are:

- All suspected drug interactions
- Reactions to any other drugs which are suspected of significantly affecting patient's management.
- Reactions suspected of causing death, life threatening conditions, hospitalization, disability, congenital anomaly.

- Reactions which involve intervention to prevent permanent impairment or damage.

Ideally the case reports must include the following details:

- Case narrative which must be precise and describe the adverse events or disease experience, including time to onset of signs or symptoms.
- Suspected and concomitant product therapy details (*i.e.* dose, frequency, lot number, regimen, dates and duration), including over the counter (OTC) medications, dietary supplements and recently discontinued medications.
- Patient characteristics including demographic information (*e.g.* age, gender, race etc), baseline medical condition prior to product therapy, co-morbid conditions, use of concomitant medications, relevant family history of disease and presence of other risk factors.
- Documentation of diagnosis of events, including methods used to make the diagnosis.
- Clinical course of the event and patients outcome (*i.e.* hospitalization, fatal or life threatening, death).
- Relevant therapeutic measures and laboratory data at baseline, during therapy and subsequent to therapy, including blood pressure etc, as appropriate.
- Information related to response with regard to rechallenge and dechallenge.
- Any other relevant information, including details which may be important in assessment of the case.

CLASSIFICATION OF ADVERSE REACTIONS

Adverse drug reactions can be categorised in a number of ways (*e.g.* by severity, by body systems affected, or by frequency). Considering the scope of this book, for simplicity purpose for the benefit of our readers, the following categorisation which is often used is enlisted:

- ***Type A*** (augmented) reactions are considered to be an exaggeration of the medicine's normal effect when given at the usual dose. This is the commonest and includes upto 80% of such reactions. They are dose dependent *i.e.*, severity increases with dose. This category includes unwanted reactions that are predictable from the drug's pharmacology and are usually dose-dependent (*e.g.,* respiratory depression with opioids and bleeding with warfarin). It is preventable in most part, by slow introduction of low dosages. Predictable by the pharmacological mechanisms, *e.g.*, hypotension by beta-blockers, hypoglycaemia caused by insulins or oral hypoglycaemics, or NSAID induced gastric ulcers.

- ***Type B*** (bizarre) reactions are effects that are not pharmacologically predictable and can include hypersensitivity reactions (*e.g.,* anaphylaxis with beta-lactam antibiotics). They are rare, idiosyncratic, genetically determined, and unpredictable. The mechanisms of such reactions are unknown, serious, and can be fatal. They are unrelated to the dose, *e.g.*, hepatitis caused by halothane, aplastic anaemia caused by chloramphenicol, neuroleptic malignant syndrome caused by some anaesthetics and antipsychotics.

Additional categories have been proposed, some to accommodate the time course of the reaction:

- ***Type C*** (continuing) reactions describe those that persist for a relatively long time (*e.g.,* osteonecrosis of the jaw with bisphosphonates). These type of reactions occur as a result of continuous drug use. They may be irreversible, unexpected, unpredictable, *e.g.* tardive dyskinesias by antipsychotics, dementia by anticholinergic medications.
- ***Type D*** (delayed) reactions, which become apparent some time after the use of a medicine (*e.g.*, leucopenia, which can occur up to 6 weeks after a dose of lomustine). Thus they depict delayed occurrence of ADRs. This could happen even after the cessation of treatment, *e.g.*, corneal opacities after thioridazine, ophthalmopathy after chloroquine, or pulmonary/peritoneal fibrosis by methyserzide.
- ***Type E (end of use):*** They are withdrawal reactions and are associated with the withdrawal of a medicine (*e.g.,* insomnia, anxiety and perceptual disturbances following withdrawal of benzodiazepines). These occur typically with the depressant drugs, *e.g.*, hypertension and restlessness in opiate abstainer, seizures on alcohol or benzodiazepines withdrawal; first dose hypotension caused by alpha-blockers (Prazosin) or ACE inhibitors.

- ***Type-F (Failure of therapy):*** Results from the ineffective treatment (previously excluded from analysis according to WHO definition), *e.g.*, accelerated hypertension because of inefficient control.

The alphabetical categories can be extended even further: Type G (genetic/genomic), Type H (hypersensitivity). The type A/type B classification of adverse drug reactions, while widely cited, does not characterise all reactions effectively. Classification along multiple axes—dose-relatedness, time-relatedness and susceptibility (DoTS)—overcomes many of the difficulties.

For simplicity we shall focus on the Rawlins and Thompson classification of adverse drug reactions. This system of classification divides adverse drug reactions into two types:

1. Type A (pharmacological)
2. Type B (idiosyncratic).

Type A reactions as discussed earlier represent an augmentation of the known pharmacological actions of a drug. These are dose-dependent and are readily reversible on dechallenge (*i.e.* on drug withdrawal) or even just after dose reduction. 80% of the adverse drug reactions belong to the category of type A reactions. On the other side, the Type B, or idiosyncratic adverse reactions, are bizarre and cannot be predicted from the known pharmacological actions of the drug. They do not elicit dose dependency and cannot be reproduced in animal models. However, these are less common than the Type A reactions. Although they cause a great deal of morbidity, in general, Type A reactions are comparatively less severe and less likely to result in fatalities than type B reactions. The differences between Type A and Type B reactions are depicted in the Table 2.

TYPE A OR PHARMACOLOGICAL ADRS

They are the most common forms of drug toxicity. Three major causes which lead to Type A ADRs are listed below:

1. Primary and secondary pharmacological characteristics of the drug

Table 2: Difference between Type A and Type B reactions

Type A reactions	*Type B reactions*
These are dose dependent reactions usually and show a good relation with dose of the drug administered.	In these reactions, the relationship with the drug dose is not simple.
These are predictable from known pharmacology.	These are not usually predictable from the known pharmacology.
Type A reactions may be dependent on host factors like genetic factors which may be important	Type B reactions are dependent usually on uncharacterised host factors.
These reactions are frequent and common	These reactions are uncommon
The severity of such reactions may vary but they are mild reactions.	The severity of such reactions may vary but they are more severe than Type B
The morbidity factor is high in such reactions but the mortality is low	The morbidity and mortality factor, both are high in such reactions.
80% of Adverse Drug Reactions are Type A	20% of Adverse Drug Reactions are Type B
First detection of Type A happens during Phase I to III of clinical trials	First detection of Type A happens during Phase IV usually but occassionally Phase III
Thus there is an early detection in Type A reactions	Thus there is a late detection in Type B reactions
The mechanism is more often due to the parent drug or stable metabolite	The mechanism may be due to the parent drug or stable metabolite
Type A reactions are usually reproducible in animal models	Type B reactions are rarely reproducible in animal models

2. Genetic polymorphism
3. Polytherapy

These are discussed in detail below.

1. ***Primary and secondary pharmacological*** characteristics of the drug are main causes for Type A reactions to occur. Thus, the secondary pharmacology of new drugs is assessed thoroughly during preclinical evaluation, to anticipate and thus avoid problems that might arise once the drug is introduced into humans.

For instance in case of fialuridine, an experimental drug for hepatitis B, 5 of 15 patients died during phase II trials whereas two others required emergency live transplants. Thus this spurred in the need for developing appropriate *in vivo* and bridging *in vitro* test systems for the prediction of secondary pharmacological adverse effects in humans. *In vitro* studies in cultured hepatoblasts have shown that the toxicity is because of the inhibition of DNA polymerase by fialuridine and its metabolites leading to mtDNA depletion and mitochondrial ultrastructural defects. Factors predisposing to pharmacological adverse reactions include dose, pharmaceutical variation in drug formulation, pharmacokinetic or pharmacodynamic abnormalities and drug–drug interactions. In essence, type A reactions occur when the drug concentration in plasma or tissue exceeds the perceived therapeutic window. Alternatively, the drug concentration may be within the normal range defined for the population, but because of increased sensitivity of the target in the individual, an adverse reaction results.

Captopril is one such example where the drug introduced into clinical practice at a particular dose was subsequently seen to be associated with an unacceptable frequency of ADRs, and for which a lower dose was found to be both safe and effective. An individual affected by a type A adverse reaction will have impairment of clearance or increased sensitivity because of the normal process of ageing, disease, concomitant drugs or genetic variation or a combination of these factors.

2. ***Genetic polymorphisms*** are also a source of variation to drug response in the human body. Genetic polymorphisms are said to be existing in a gene, if the variant allele exists in the normal population at a frequency of atleast 1%. Polymorphisms in both pharmacokinetic and pharmacodynamic parameters can act as predisposing factors in case of Type A ADRs. Genetically mediated deficiencies of the drug-metabolising enzymes are one such example of genetic polymorphism. Further when such genetically modified enzyme metabolises the drug, it shows an increased half life due to reduced elimination from the body, thus eliciting a dose-dependent toxicity.

Some of the examples are cited below where there is an observation of genetic polymorphism:

A. Neutropenia with azathioprine in patients deficient in the enzyme thiopurine methyltransferase is one such example.

B. Yet another example is CYP2C9 genetic variation is the metabolism of warfarin. Warfarin is the oral anticoagulant of choice in the United Kingdom and largely so because of its use in atrial fibrillation. CYP2C9 metabolises the S-enantiomer of warfarin, which is predominantly responsible for the anticoagulant effect. Reducing the risk of bleeding depends on accurate dosage regimen during warfarin therapy. Because of the genetic polymorphism, warfarin runs the risk of haemorrhage. This is observed in case of 8–26 per 100 patient and is related to the intensity of anticoagulation. Predicting accurate dosages for patients during warfarin therapy however is difficult because there is 20-fold interindividual variability in the dose. Polymorphisms in the CYP2C9 gene result in at least two allelic variants, CYP2C9*2 _Arg144 →Cys_ and CYP2C9*3 _Ile359→Leu_. Both these alleles have been responsible to decrease warfarin clearance *in vitro* and *in vivo*.

These variants have shown the below mentioned three effects:

a. Reduced warfarin dose requirement,

b. Greater difficulty in initiating warfarin treatment and

c. An increased risk of bleeding.

Albeit, the association of CYP2C9 genotype with respect to warfarin-related bleeding is observed but the association is not as strong as that observed with dose.

Vitamin K epoxide reductase complex 1 (VKORC1) is the target for the action of warfarin. Polymorphism in vitamin K epoxide reductase complex 1 (VKORC1) determine dose requirement of warfarin. The effect of VKORC1 seems to be quantitatively greater than that of CYP2C9. Whether such genotype-based dosing, in the absence of other possible factors that might influence dose requirements, including drug interactions, diet, underlying disease, *e.g.* thyroid disease, and polymorphisms in other genes involved in the mode of action of warfarin, will lead to an improvement in the dosing and safety of warfarin, needs to be further probed.

3. ***Polytherapy / Drug*** interaction is yet another reason which is the major cause of Type A reactions. As the number of drugs prescribed

increases the probability of developing an adverse reaction increases. Thus polytherapy is directly proportional to adverse drug reaction. It was noted in an Australian study that 4.4% of all ADRs resulting in hospital admission were because of drug interactions, whereas a study in the United Kingdom showed that one in six of all adverse reactions causing hospital admission were because of interactions. Enzyme induction and Enzyme inhibition are two factors which may lead to altered/modified metabolism of drugs. When Enzyme induction happens, it lead to increased metabolism of the drug and the drug clearance increases proportionally. This will lead to reduced drug efficacy rather than drug toxicity (unless the adverse reaction is because of a metabolite rather than the parent drug). On the other hand, Enzyme inhibition is more likely to lead to type A ADRs and have been instrumental in regulatory action in many instances. This is owing to the fact that the clearance of the affected drug is reduced; this is particularly likely when the affected drug has a narrow therapeutic index.

Especially in the geriatric population where administering many drugs at a time or in a day/polypharmacy is prevalent, ADRs are more prominent. Increase in the ADRs is also the case with younger patients having chronic diseases such as AIDS, where patients may be on 6–10 different drugs.

Some examples are cited below which has shown ADRS due to Polypharmacy:

A. The interaction between CYP3A4 inhibitors ketoconazole and erythromycin and the non-sedating antihistamine terfenadine shows ADR due to unconverted Terfenadine. The interaction resulted in decreased conversion of terfenadine to its active metabolite (now marketed as fexofenadine). Terfenadine blood concentrations affects the delayed rectifier potassium current, which results in the prolongation of QT interval, torsades de pointes and sudden death.

B. An interaction between cisapride and CYP3A4 inhibitors has also resulted in regulatory action against cisapride.

C. Interactions due to natural foods such as grapefruit juice and cranberry juice are also a causal factor for ADRs.

D. Drug transporters in the disposition of drugs are another cause for ADRs. Many drug transport proteins are present on membranes, some of which are responsible for drug influx and efflux and some which can transport in both directions. Overexpression of P-glycoprotein (Pgp) (which is encoded by the multi-drug resistance 1 (MDR1) gene), is one of the mechanisms responsible for resistance of tumours to chemotherapy. However, Pgp is also responsible for the transport of many other drugs including digoxin. Digoxin interacts with drugs such as quinidine, verapamil and amiodarone, all of which can precipitate digoxin toxicity. It in itself does not undergo any significant degree of metabolism. The mechanism of this interaction involves the inhibition of Pgp, thereby reducing efflux of digoxin from the gut and kidney. With further intensified studies on transporters and their drug substrates, it is likely that this will be identified as the mechanism underlying many adverse drug interactions

TYPE B OR IDIOSYNCRATIC ADVERSE REACTIONS

Idiosyncratic adverse reactions are responsible for many fatal ADRs and are accountable for many drug induced deaths. Even if they are less common than the pharmacological adverse reactions but they are more serious in nature. Drug hypersensitivity reactions fall into the category of type B (or bizarre) adverse drug reactions. An inappropriate immune response that leads to tissue damage from an otherwise nontoxic agent is hypersensitivity. Thus, these reactions cannot be predicted from the known pharmacology of the drug and do not show a simple dose-response relationship.

We shall see the influence of the following factors on Type B or idiosyncratic reactions, which are as mentioned below:

1. Dose of the drug administered
2. Role of Metabolism
3. Role of Immune system
4. Role of Genetic predisposition
5. Role of Viruses

1. ***Dose of the drug administered:*** They are not dose dependent and hence there is no relationship between dose and the occurrence of toxicity. In case of hypersensitive patients, the doses of the drug

administered are lower since the drug had to be withdrawn and also the relationship between the occurrence of toxicity and the dose administered is very modest. Hence if we take into consideration the patients who are and not hypersensitive to a particular drug, they actually project a very little difference in the doses of the drug received. However it must be noted that the hypersensitive reaction is triggered because of atleast a trace amount or dose of drug entering the systemic circulation of the patient. This goes on to say that there is definitely some kind of dose response relationship between the drug and the ADR, because if the patient had not received the drug then he would not have developed the hypersensitivity reaction in the first place. Also the ADRs may affect many organ systems either in isolation or in combination. Formation of Chemically reactive metabolites (CRMs) through P450 enzymes are triggarants to many of the Type B ADRs. Thus the concentration of toxic metabolites in the body sets off this process of bioactivation leading to ADRs.

However, the dose-response relationship assessment has been rather difficult because of the unstable nature of metabolites. Also the dose response relationship would vary because of the different sources of variation in human body.

For instance, this example details about different sources of variations in human body and pursuant relationship between dose responses of the drug administered. Low doses of co-trimoxazole is given for prophylaxis against Pneumocystis carinii pneumonia (PCP) (960 mg once daily) in HIV positive patients whereas for acute treatment of PCP, higher doses upto 8 g/day needs to be given. Also the rate at which hypersensitivity reactions occur with prophylactic dose (30%) is lower than with the acute dose, where rates as high as 80% have been reported. Thus it can be seen that in real clinical situations different doses have to be given to the same group of patient in different circumstances.

2. ***Role of drug metabolism:*** This plays a significant role in precipitating Type B reactions. The drug bioactivation and bioinactivation process imbalance may lead to an inadequate toxication of CRM which often leads to idiosyncratic drug toxicity. This is discussed in detail below. A drug metabolising enzyme such as Phase I and/or II is required for the drug metabolising process

which is detoxication process. In the process the drug undergoes either Phase I and II metabolism or Phase I or Phase II metabolism. This process involves the conversion of therapeutically active compounds to inactive metabolites which is excreted harmless from the body. As discussed above, the metabolism process can also include conversion of a drug to toxic CRM by the process known as bioactivation which represents less than 1% of the overall metabolism of a drug. Cytochrome P450 enzymes are majorly instrumental in bioactivation process although Phase I and II enzymes may also lead to the CRM generation process. If the amount of toxic metabolite formed is below a toxic threshold or is detoxified by the defence mechanism that body is equipped with, it does not lead to toxicity. The process known as bioinactivation refers to the detoxication of the CRM thus preventing tissue damage. An imbalance between drug bioactivation and bioinactivation process may lead to an inadequate toxication of CRM. This often leads to idiosyncratic drug toxicity. An inadequate detoxication of a CRM, although an important first step in the occurrence of toxicity, is not necessarily the ultimate step. Other factors such as tissue repair enzymes, immune responsiveness and the biochemical processes that modulate tissue injury help in assessing the severity along with identifying if idiosyncratic toxicity has occurred. An inadequately detoxified CRM can combine with or damage cellular macromolecules such as proteins and nucleic acids and result in various forms of toxicity including teratogenicity, carcinogenicity, cellular necrosis and hypersensitivity.

How these toxicities occur has been listed below:

A. The binding of a CRM to nucleic acid may result in teratogenicity or carcinogenicity.

B. The binding to cellular macromolecules may result in either direct or immune-mediated toxicity.

C. With direct toxicity, binding of the CRM to a protein will interfere with its normal physiological function leading to cellular necrosis.

D. Alternatively, the CRM can act as a hapten and initiate an immune reaction that may be because of a specific humoral (antibody) response, a cellular response (T lymphocytes) or a combination of both. The immune response can be directed against the drug (haptenic epitopes), the carrier protein (auto-antigenic determinants) or the neoantigen created by the combination of the drug and the protein (new antigenic determinants).

The factors that determine what type of toxicity is mediated by a CRM are poorly understood but are likely to include:

- the relative stability of the CRM, and thus its reactivity;
- the half-life of any drug–protein adducts that are formed and their concentration within the cell;
- the epitope density, *i.e.* the number of groups of the CRM that are covalently bound to a protein molecule; and
- the nature, physiological function and subcellular site of the carrier protein to which the CRM binds.

In most cases, the differentiation between these two forms of idiosyncratic toxicity is largely empirical being based on symptomatology; *e.g.* the occurrence of manifestations such as rash, fever, lymphadenopathy and eosinophilia all suggest drug hypersensitivity. The lack of laboratory methodology by which to make a definitive diagnosis largely reflects our ignorance of the mechanism of toxicity in most cases of idiosyncratic toxicity.

Tissue selective toxicity is triggered by selective imbalance in that tissue due to tissue specific expression of enzymes that partcipate in drug bioactivation and drug detoxication. An imbalance may be either due to genetically determined deficiency of an enzyme, or alternatively or it may be acquired because of environmental factors such as infection, diet or concomitant drug intake.

CRM induced toxicity can be best understood by an example of Paracetamol. If the drug is taken in therapeutic doses, CRMs formed will be detoxified by normal enzymatic or non-enzymatic cellular defence mechanisms. But if there is an over dosage of medicine, CRMs formed will be so large in number that it will overpower the cellular detoxication process and thereby lead to cellular damage. For many drugs that undergo metabolism, CRM will be formed irrespective of the dose of the drug. When a drug is taken in therapeutic dosage, any toxic metabolite formed will be detoxified by normal enzymatic or non-enzymatic cellular defence mechanisms. An imbalance between bioactivation and bioinactivation leading to toxicity may however be created by taking a drug overdose. This will lead to the formation of large amounts of CRM, overwhelm the cellular detoxication capacity and lead to cell damage. The classic example of this is paracetamol, which causes hepatotoxicity when taken in overdosage, and causes around 160 deaths per year in the United Kingdom. Paracetamol hepatotoxicity does not fit into the definition of ADR and thus should not be classified as an ADR, because the hepatic injury occurs when the drug is used inappropriately, *i.e.* in high doses. But, it is important to note that the occurrence of liver damage with paracetamol and its severity is a function not only of the dose but also of various other factors as well. Indeed, paracetamol hepatotoxicity has been reported with therapeutic drug use. For example, the maximum therapeutic dose of paracetamol that is recommended is 4 g/day. In a particular study, 40% of the population who had taken less than this maximum recommended dose of 4 g/day sustained liver injury. 67 alcoholics sustained liver injury after paracetamol ingestion, out of which 40% had taken less than 4 g/day (the maximum recommended therapeutic dose), whereas another 20% had taken between 4 and 6 g/day (which is also regarded as a non-toxic dose). In therapeutic dosage, paracetamol is largely metabolised by phase II processes (glucuronidation and sulphation) to stable metabolites, but between 5% and 10% also undergoes P450 metabolism to the toxic N-acetyl p-benzoquinoneimine (NAPQI) metabolite. This is detoxified by cellular glutathione. Hepatotoxicity happens due to the depletion of cellular glutathione in case of overdosage. When there is an overdose, saturation of the phase II metabolic pathways results in a greater proportion of the drug undergoing bioactivation. Also consumption of alcohol can lead to a greater susceptibility to paracetamol related hepatocellular toxicity which is explained below. This ultimately leads to the depletion of cellular glutathione and allows the toxic metabolite to bind to hepatic proteins resulting in hepatocellular damage. By studying the mechanisms of durg toxicity carefully, therapies can be developed which can prevent toxicity. The use of N-acetylcysteine in the treatment of paracetamol overdosage demonstrates the important point that explication of the mechanism of drug toxicity can lead to the development of rational therapies that will prevent the toxicity. Alcohol induces P450 isoform CYP2E1 and depletes glutathione. Hence alcoholics show increased susceptibility to paracetamol overdosage because excess alcohol consumption results in the depletion of glutathione and induction of the P450 isoform CYP2E1. It is important to understand that P450 isoform CYP2E1 actually triggers the bioactivation process in paracetamol, which means the production of toxic metabolites. Studies pertaining to knockout mice have shown that CYP2E1 is the primary isoform involved in the bioactivation of paracetamol. But in case of experiments with transgenic mice, phase I oxidative pathways were absent and thus resulted in NAPQI formation. But this did not result in hepatotoxicity in this instance. Hence the specific pathway leading to liver damage is still unclear. Quite a few mechanisms depict the effects on plasma membrane Ca^{2+} pumps, which can lead to Ca^{2+}- induced DNA damage, mitochondrial damage resulting in glutathione depletion and oxidative stress and apoptosis. Also some studies reveal that Fas antisense oligonucleotide protects mice from paracetamol toxicity, which goes on to say that the ultimate cytotoxic event involves more than simply necrosis and that cells of the immune system may play a significant role in the inflammatory response.

Studies have revealed that when cells are exposed to chemical or oxidant stress, they respond with a vigorous and forceful transcriptional response that is designed at detoxifying the offending chemical and preventing or repairing cellular damage. If this is unsuccessful, then the conclusion of this reaction is to commit the cell to suicide through apoptosis. The target genes for the antioxidant response encode a set of enzymes and other proteins that scavenge or search for free radicals, neutralise electrophiles or up-regulate the critical cellular thiol, glutathione. Glutathione depletion caused by a range of chemicals leads to the up-regulation of c-jun and c-fos Mrna and enhances activator protein-1 (AP-1) DNA binding activity. This response was also accompanied by the induction of _ glutamyl cysteine synthetase (GCS).

Another important mechanism of cell protection involves the nuclear translocation of redox-sensitive transcription factors such as Nrf-2, which 'sense' chemical danger and coordinate cell defence. Importantly, it has been observed that nuclear translocation occurs at non-toxic doses of paracetamol and before explicit toxicity is observed. However, with increasing doses of acetaminophen, there is progressive dislocation of nuclear translocation, transcription, translation and protein activity as the rate of drug bioactivation overpowers cell defence through the destruction of critical proteins – at least 31 of these critical proteins have been identified. Ironically, studies performed with transgenic mice aimed at clarifying events subsequent to NAPQI formation have only served to confound rather than to clarify. For example, the removal of components of the glutathione detoxication system such as glutathione peroxidase and glutathione transferase-pi (GST-pi) both gave incomplete protection against paracetamol hepatotoxicity. A reduction in the glutathione conjugation of NAPQI due to the loss of a major hepatic form of GST, which represents over 3% of total soluble protein would have predisposed the animals to hepatotoxicity. This suggests that GST-pi may be involved in a novel mechanism that determines susceptibility to paracetamol hepatotoxicity. Also, a recent study has shown that GST-pi may have a role in cell signaling; wherein it was seen to be an efficient inhibitor of Jun kinase (also known as stress-activated kinase), the enzyme that activates cjun and several other transcription factors. Future studies using other transgenic mouse models will be useful in determining the exact pathway by which paracetamol causes liver damage and may therefore provide novel therapeutic strategies by which to reverse liver damage after paracetamol overdosage.

3. ***Role of immune system:*** Hapten hypothesis explains the immune mediated adverse reactions caused by a specific drug. Evidences suggest that quite a few idiosyncratic or Type B reactions are caused due to an immune mediation process.

   There are various type of signals to present an immunogenic reaction, they are:

   A. The term 'hapten' has been coined to describe such substances that are not immunogenic *per se* but become immunogenic when conjugated to a macromolecular carrier (this has been termed 'signal 1').

   B. Signal 2 is represented by a series of proinflammatory cytokines such as interleukin-2 (IL-2), TNF-_ and IFN-_ that act indirectly on antigen presenting cells to up-regulate the expression of costimulatory molecules.

C. Signal 3 represents polarizing cytokines that act directly on T cells. It is known that TH1 cells produce IL-12 and IFN-_, which promote the activation of macrophages and cell mediated immunity.

In addition to signal 1, signal 2 and signal 3 are required to stimulate a full immune response. The fundamental concept of protein conjugation required for immune recognition as in case of signal 1 has been challenged. This is explained in further detail with an example related to T cell clones. Hapten hypothesis makes an assumption that small molecules such as drugs (<1000 Da) can be recognised as immunogens (*i.e.* a substance capable of eliciting a specific immune response) only when they become covalently bound to an autologous high molecular weight (>50 000 Da) macromolecular carrier such as a protein. The site of antigen formation and the immune response determines the type of hypersensitive reaction.

For *e.g.*: Penicillins and cephalosporins show Type I hypersensitivity reaction and are mediated by immunoglobulin E (IgE) antibodies directed against a drug hapten conjugated to protein. Severe anaphylactic reactions occur in only few patients (1 in 2000) and atopic patients are at increased risk. The IgE response to penicillins and genetic implication remains to be elucidated. Skin reactions such as Stevens–Johnson syndrome (SJS) and immunoallergic hepatitis are yet not clearly understood. The immune mechanisms pertaining to these reactions needs to be further studied and analysed. *In vitro* studies suggest that the drugs associated with these reactions can undergo oxidative metabolism to CRMs. The CRMs further haptenate proteins. In addition, both humoral and cell-mediated responses directed against drug induced antigen have been detected in patients, *e.g.* in halothane hepatitis. The immune reactions by auto antibodies have been explained with an example of Tienilic acid. In tienilic acid-induced hepatitis, patients have circulating auto-antibodies directed against the P450 isoform (CYP2C9), which is responsible for the bioactivation of tienilic acid. This further leads to the formation of CRMs.

T-cell clones from patients hypersensitive to many drugs undergo proliferation in an antigen processing–independent but major histocompatibility complex (MHC)-restricted manner. Thus this goes ahead to explain that protein conjugation is not an obligatory step in the process of immune recognition. This process involves reversible binding of drug to the MHC complexes on antigen-presenting cells. This mechanism thus represents the proliferation of T-cell clones only in response to parent drug rather than metabolite and the rapid down-regulation in expression of the T-cell receptor upon stimulation. Both mechanisms *i.e.* hapten dependent pathway and metabolism independent pathway may be important in the overall pathogenesis. One leads to primary stimulation and the other leads to secondary stimulation. For primary immune stimulation or sensitization, the hapten dependent pathway may be more important, whereas for secondary stimulation the metabolism-independent pathway may be all that is necessary. Of course the roles of two pathways of drug (antigen) presentation in the pathogenesis of immune mediated Adverse Drug Reactions needs further probing.

The immune response is governed by the interaction between the T cell and the drug (antigen) in the groove of the MHC. T cells are of fundamental importance in the immune response against a drug whatever might be the way of antigen presentation. The two types of MHC class molecules are listed below:

A. MHC class I molecules bind peptides of 8–10 amino acids and present to CD^{8+} T cells. Class I molecules are found on all cell surfaces

B. MHC class II molecules present longer peptide molecules (13–17 amino acids) to CD^{4+} cells. Class II molecules are only expressed on specialised antigen presenting cells such as macrophages but can become expressed on other cells such as keratinocytes in the presence of pro-inflammatory cytokines such as interferon-gamma (INF-_).

The nature of the immune response is governed by the differentiation of T cells into T-helper 1 _TH1__ TH2, T-cytotoxic 1 _TC1_ or TC2 subsets. TH1 and TC1 cells mediate cytotoxicity and local inflammatory reactions, whereas TH2 and TC2 cells stimulate B-cell-dependent antibody production. It is important to note that the presence of an antigen (*i.e.* signal 1) in the absence of co-stimulatory molecules will lead to tolerance and T-cell apoptosis. Co-stimulatory molecules are B7.1 and B7.2 and cytokines. Also another hypothesis such as 'danger hypothesis' explains the basis of self tolerance. The danger hypothesis states that only in the presence of a danger signal will the presentation of an antigen result in an immune response otherwise the immune system responds to most antigens with tolerance. The potential candidates for danger signals are pro-inflammatory and polarising cytokines, intracellular contents resulting from cell necrosis and exogenous proteins including those derived from viruses, are all potential candidates. This can also be applied to the mechanism of drug hypersensitivity. With respect to drug hypersensitivity, it can be hypothesised that the CRM may not only provide signal 1 (by conjugating with a protein) but also provide the co-stimulatory signals 2 and 3 by the activation of signalling pathways linked to oxidative stress and protein damage, including the secretion of cytokines.

4. ***The role of viruses In type B adverse drug reactions:*** A patient who has concomitant virus infections, is quite likely to develop idiosyncratic ADRs, particularly the ones that are thought to be immune mediated. In this case the source of danger signal is the viruses leading to the Type B or Idiosyncratic reactions.

   For instance, First discovery of role of viruses in developing idiosyncratic reactions occurred when patients with active Epstein–Barr virus (EBV) infection (*i.e.* infectious mononucleosis) were given ampicillin. It was observed in this particular case that 95% of patients developed rashes as a result of presence of viruse Epstein–Barr virus (EBV). Another example is of the human herpes virus 6 (HHV6) which leads to hypersensitivity reactions associated with many drugs including sulphasalazine. But definitely further studies needs to be conducted to confirm the role of viruses in such reactions or if the occurrence was a sheer coincidence. Thus the suspected causality needs to be transformed in to a confirmed causality. Yet another example is of viral infection and drug hypersensitivity which has been observed in HIV (Human Immuno Deficiency Virus)-infected individuals. These patients have a higher frequency of hypersensitivity reactions with numerous anti-infective drugs including co-trimoxazole, sulphadiazine, dapsone, clindamycin, primaquine and thioacetazone. The increased susceptibility of HIV patients to Idiosyncratic reactions can be explained with the example of co-trimoxazole that is used for the treatment of PCP.

Skin rashes developed in around 50% of patients being treated acutely for PCP whereas approximately 30% of patients who consumed co-trimoxazole developed the same when used for prophylaxis. On the other hand only 3% developed skin rashes in case of HIV-negative individuals. There is yet another inference that can be drawn apart from Viruses resposnsible for causing Type B ADRs that is obvious from the fact that only 3% of the population developed skin rashes who were HIV negative. The inference being also the dose of the drug that is consumed may lead to Type B ADR. This is evident from the fact that 50% developed rashes by an acute treatment and only 30% developed rashes from prophylactic treatment with co-trimoxazole. This can be further elaborated from the information that HIV population is deficient for thiols such as glutathione and cysteine. The drug sulphamethoxazole produces a toxic substance called nitroso on metabolism. However this is detoxified by the presence of plasma cysteine. But in case of HIV patients due to deficiency of cysteine, the nitroso concentrations increase in plasma which leads to idiosyncratic reactions. And if increased dose of sulphamethoxazole is given to a HIV patient, then it may lead to more production of nitroso and thereby increasing the intensity of Type B ADRs. Also a prophylactic use of N-acetylcysteine, was unable to prevent co-trimoxazole hypersensitivity.

Also a prophylactic use of N-acetylcysteine, was unable to prevent co-trimoxazole hypersensitivity. N-acetylcysteine was given to HIV patients with an expectation that the increased cysteine levels would reduce the idiosyncratic reactions. But this was not the case observed, suggesting that there are other factors which contribute to idiosyncratic reactions in HIV positive patients:

A. The dose of the drug as already discussed above.

B. Changes in drug metabolising capacity (both in bioactivation and in bioinactivation). This means the metabolism rate and the rate at which the toxic metabolites are detoxified.

C. *Immune dysregulation:* With the new antiretrovirals such as abacavir and non nucleoside reverse transcriptase inhibitors such as nevirapine, efavirenz and delavirdine coming into market, they too seem to be associated with severe hypersensitivity reactions.

5. ***Role of genetic predisposition:*** Genes have long since been suspected for Type B ADRs and now there are many novel genes which are likely to be identified as predisposing factors for hypersensitivity reactions in the near future. Every individual possessing a unique genetic makeup will have differing Idiosyncratic reactions to the drug concerned. If we are going to connect genetics with the ADRs, then there are two ways to do this:

   A. *Multigenic:* As the name suggests, the ADRs would be linked to a combination of genes.

   B. *Multifactorial:* ADRs that are linked to an interaction between genetic and environmental factors.

The multiple gene inclination for ADRs could be divided into several areas as follows:

1. ***Drug activation***
2. ***Drug bioinactivation***
3. ***Immune response genes***
4. ***Tissue injury genes***

1. ***Drug activation:*** This relates to the activation of drug to chemically reactive metabolites (CRMs). This process known as bioactivation of drugs is largely mediated by cytochrome P450 enzymes, many of which have now been shown to be polymorphically expressed. Thus an augmentation of cytochrome P450 due to polygenic factors will lead to increased bioactivation. Importantly, a deficiency of an enzyme will lead to reduced bioactivation of a drug and will act as a protective factor, as the CRM level will be decreased.

2. ***Drug bioinactivation:*** This is the process of detoxifying the chemically reactive metabolite. This process of detoxification of reactive metabolites by detoxifying enzymes to inactive substances is known as boinactivation, which occurs via accumulation or binding to humoral and cellular proteins. A deficiency of these detoxifying enzymes would lead to an increase in the chemically reactive metabolites by decrement in bioinactivation process. The CRMs in turn interact with the celluar macromolecules and lead to varios forms of toxicity. Glutathione-S-transferase genes have been shown to be polymorphically expressed. A deficiency of this

enzyme may lead to decreased bioinactivation causing toxicity or ADRs. Many cancer drugs show Idiosyncratic reactions due to genetic polymorphism.

3. ***Immune-response genes:*** When a drug/drug metabolite is recognized as being foreign or antigenic by the bodys' natural immune system, the body responds to it by the mechanism of an immune response and is perceived as a defence mechanism. But the same may also be lead to hypersensitivity reactions. MHC, co-stimulatory molecules and T cell receptor are examples of gene encoding for immune responsiveness.
4. ***Tissue-injury genes:*** The process by which an immune response is translated into tissue injury, the nature and extent of which can be counteracted by repair mechanisms that limit any tissue damage. Representative candidates include cytokines, chemokines and prostaglandins. MHC seems to play a major role in the genetic predisposition to drug hypersensitivity. These are illustrated below with reference to two compounds, abacavir and CBZ.

Major histocompatibility complex (MHC) is a large cluster of genes found on the short arm of chromosome 6. Many of the genes in this complex play significant roles in the immune system. MHC is categorized into three classes, viz: Class I, II and III. Class I and II MHC genes encode human leukocyte antigens (HLAs), proteins that are displayed on cell surface and define an individuals' tissue type. Everyone's immune system is tolerant of its own HLAs, but if foreign HLAs are detected then the cells displaying them are destroyed. Class I is found virtually on all cell types. Class II is seen only on immune cells. Class III MHC genes encode many components of the complement system, a assortment of soluble proteins found in the blood that targets foreign cells and breaks open their membranes. MHC depicts a high degree of polymorphism (100 times higher than the genome average *i.e.* a 10 percent difference between any two unrelated individuals). Many of these polymorphisms are associated with either amplified or diminished susceptibility to a series of infectious diseases including malaria, tuberculosis, leprosy, typhoid fever, hepatitis and HIV/AIDS.

E.g.: Abacavirs' use as a potent HIV-1 reverse transcriptase inhibitor, has been impeded by the occurrence of hypersensitivity reaction in approximately 5% of patients. These reactions are characterized by skin rashes and gastrointestinal and respiratory manifestations and can occasionally be fatal, particularly on rechallenge. A strong connection is established between abacavir hypersensitivity and the halotype comprising HLA-B*5701, HLADR7 and HLA DQ3 with an odds ratio of over 100. The same association however has not been shown in an African American population presumably because of ethnic differences in linkage disequilibrium patterns in the MHC. The association with the MHC in whites is consistent with the immune nature of the reaction and the identification of drug specific T cells in abacavir hypersensitive patients. By contrast, no association has been found with polymorphisms in the genes coding for various abacavir-metabolising enzymes. In whites genotyping for HLA-B*5701 should be executed before the prescription of abacavir, and this has resulted in a decline in the incidence of abacavir hypersensitivity. An examination of the cost effectiveness of prospective HLAB*5701 genotyping, demonstrated that in whites this would be a cost-effective strategy.

Carbamazepine Hypersensitivity; Carbamazepine, a widely used anticonvulsant, causes rashes in up to 10% of patients, and in occasional cases, this may be the precursor to the progress of a hypersensitivity syndrome characterised by systemic manifestations such as fever and eosinophilia. Sometimes, CBZ can stimulate blistering skin reactions such as SJS and toxic epidermal necrolysis, two conditions associated with a high fatality rate. CBZ hypersensitivity is a T-cell-mediated disease. CBZ is metabolised to CRMs that have been implicated in the pathogenesis of hypersensitivity. Till date, no polymorphisms in the drug metabolising enzyme gene polymorphisms have been associated with susceptibility to CBZ hypersensitivity. MHC analysis reveals that CBZ hypersensitivity syndrome and not mild maculopapular eruptions, is associated with the haplotype TNF2-DR3-DQ2. These studies suggest that in whites the causal variant for CBZ hypersensitivity resides on the ancestral haplotype 8.1. In the Han Chinese, a strong association was observed between CBZ-induced SJS and HLA-B*1502. SNP maps may be used to screen for pharmacogenetically active genes as whole genome. SNPs are single-base differences in the DNA sequence, observed between individuals, which occur throughout the human genome. High-density SNP maps will provide an opportunity to perform SNP profiling to identify genetic factors predisposing to ADRs.

The importance of ADRs is often underestimated. They are common, can be life threatening and unnecessarily expensive. Because of plethora of drugs available with varying mechanisms of action, the manifestations of toxicity can be unpredictable and affect any organ system. Besides, the pattern of toxicity is going to change with the introduction of new biotechnology products. It is therefore important for the prescribing clinician to be aware of the toxic profile of drugs they prescribe and to be wary for the incidence of unexpected adverse reactions. Both type A and type B adverse reactions are complex and intricate, and their deterrence for future generation will depend on an understanding of their pathogenesis and exactly how a foreign chemical, *i.e.* drug, interacts with macromolecules within the body. Pharmacogenomic strategies have been proposed and inspite of the propaganda there is all likelihood that this will be a long-term goal and will depend on (a) the availability of accurately phenotyped patients, which for the rare reactions will necessitate multi-centre international collaborations; (b) the demonstration that genotyping is clinical and cost-effective; (c) an understanding of the mechanisms of the adverse reactions so that more targeted SNP profiling can be undertaken and (d) educating of the clinicians, so that they understand the rationale for performing the tests and how to interpret the results.

Thus understanding the safety of medicines will encourage striking a balance between the benefits and harms of medicines which will result in an integrated approach to therapeutic decision-making. Excessive and irrational drug use contributes to adverse reactions which are due to the poor quality and inaccessibility of drug information available to practitioners. These problems are worsened by:

- Aggressive and inaccurate marketing and advertising
- Uninformed patient use and their demands for the latest medicines
- Lack of accurate drug information.

Indicators of inappropriate drug use can be procured from spontaneous reports of ADRs. Case studies may serve as useful teaching tools for improving the safe use of medicines. Medication errors and ADRs are well known in hospitalized and non-hospitalized patients, and they contribute considerably to morbidity and mortality. They also contribute to the number of hospital admissions and are known to occur in the community setting. Many of the ADR's being predictable and preventable, suggests considerable opportunity for minimizing the risks of ADRs through rational use, monitoring and follow-up. Early detection is important, particularly in hospitals where systems for detecting ADRs and medication errors will save lives and money. Prospective hospital-based surveillance minimizes the risk and severity of ADRs. There is further, a need to provide health care professionals with the skills required to assess drug information critically and to decide how the safety profile of a drug (*e.g.* developed from population data) might be applied to a particular patient. Often, the manufacturer's product information and promotional materials are the only information available to the practitioner and evidence-based, comprehensive sources may not be available. Availability of balanced and reliable drug information is likely to improve standards of use and to reduce the occurrence of adverse reactions. Information that includes patients' subjective experiences of adverse reactions would be beneficial to patients and to prescribers of medicines. Product safety information often consists of lists of adverse reactions, rated in order of frequency, without real description of how these might affect quality of life. Research in ADRs and pharmaco-epidemiology in departments of internal medicine and pharmacology should be encouraged and promoted. In the training of health professionals it is important to build up proficiency in evaluating and communicating information about benefit, harm, effectiveness and risk to the patient.

4

Causality Assessment

A structured and harmonised system of causality assessment is essential, because case reports are more often suspected adverse drug reactions. Thus ensuring causal relation between the drug and the adverse reaction is an inherent problem associated with Pharmacovigilance studies. A rechallenge of the drug in case of adverse drug reaction is rarely justified and diagnostic tests are recurrently absent. Very few adverse reactions are certain or unlikely, most of them fall into the category of possible or probable. Of the many systems developed, none of them are actually capable of producing a precise or reliable quantitative estimation of the relationship likelihod between the drug and adverse reaction.

The WHO UMC system for International Drug monitoring is a practical tool for the assessment of case reports. It is combined assessment taking into account the clinical/pharmacological aspects of the case history and the quality of documentation of the observation. Statistical chance and previous knowledge plays rather a lesser significant role because pharmacovigilance is about detection of the unknown and unexpected adverse drug reaction. A standard basis of categorizing the observed events, their laboratory value assessment, response to withdrawal, time relationship of the event with drug intake is done taking into consideration some parameters which are discussed in detail in the Table 1.

Table 1: Assessment criteria of various causality terms

Causality term	***Assessment criteria***	***Rechallenge/ Dechallenge***
Certain	• Event or laboratory test abnormality, with plausible time relationship to drug intake • Cannot be explained by disease or other drugs • Response to withdrawal plausible (pharmacologically, pathologically) • Event definitive pharmacologically or phenomenologically (*i.e.* an objective and specific medical disorder or a recognized pharmacological phenomenon)	Rechallenge satisfactory, if necessary
Probable/ Likely	Event or laboratory test abnormality, with reasonable time relationship to drug intake • Unlikely to be attributed to disease or other drugs • Response to withdrawal clinically reasonable.	Rechallenge not required
Possible	Event or laboratory test abnormality, with reasonable time relationship to drug intake • Could also be explained by disease or other drugs • Information on drug withdrawal may be lacking or unclear.	
Unlikely	• Event or laboratory test abnormality, with a time to drug intake that makes a relationship improbable (but not impossible). • Disease or other drugs provide plausible explanations.	
Conditional/ Unclassified	Event or laboratory test abnormality • More data for proper assessment needed, or • Additional data under examination	
Unassessable/ Unclassifiable	• Report suggesting an adverse reaction • Cannot be judged because information is insufficient or contradictory • Data cannot be supplemented or verified	

The certain criteria includes, a clinical event, including laboratory test abnormality, occurring in a plausible time relationship after drug administration. The event which has occurred must be such that, it cannot be explained by concurrent disease or other drugs or chemicals. On drug withdrawal *i.e.*, dechallenge, the response should be clinically plausible. Likewise, by means of a satisfactory rechallenge procedure if necessary, the event must be definitive pharmacologically or phenomenologically. Thus, as observed this stringent definition of the criteria "Certain" will lead to very few reports matching the criteria. What needs to be taken care in case of such assessments is that, apart from time relationship of the event (onset and course) with regards to drug administration, due weight and emphasis must also be laid on pharmacological and other characteristics of the drug product. Occasionally there are cases, for instance, penicillin anaphylaxis, where the clinical phenomena in itself is self-sufficient for a confident causality analysis. This assessment is possible even if relevant confounding features or apt time relationships are missing to the case. For 'Certain', rechallenge information with a satisfactory outcome is requested (*i.e.* what has happened when the drug was first stopped and later on resumed), unless the evidence in the report is already convincing without a re-exposure.

In case of Probable, it is a clinical event, including laboratory test abnormality, with a reasonable time sequence to administration of the drug, unlikely to be attributed to concurrent disease or other drugs or chemicals, and which follows a clinically reasonable response on withdrawal (dechallenge). Thus the definition of probable has less stringent wording than for "certain" and does not necessitate prior knowledge of drug characteristics or clinical adverse reaction phenomena. Rechallenge information is not required to fulfil this definition. To qualify as 'Certain' the interval between the start of the drug and the onset of the event must be 'plausible'; this means that there is sufficient detail to support the view that the drug is causally involved, pharmacologically or pathologically. For 'Probable' the time relationship should be 'reasonable'; this is a more neutral term covering everything that is not unreasonable. As stated no rechallenge information is needed in case of "Probable", but confounding drug administration underlying disease must be absent.

Further, for 'Certain' the occurrence of the event cannot be explained by any disease the patient is known to have or any other drug taken. For 'Probable', on the other hand, the event is 'unlikely' to be attributable to another cause. Also the dechallenge situations (*i.e.* what happened after stopping) are different. In a 'Certain' case report, the course of events constitutes a positive argument in favour of holding the suspected drug responsible, in pharmacological or pathological respects, whereas in a 'Probable' case it is sufficient if it is 'clinically reasonable' (*i.e.* not unreasonable).

In case of Possible, it is a clinical event, including laboratory test abnormality, with a reasonable time sequence to administration of the drug. This type of an event could also be explained by concurrent disease or other drugs or chemicals. This definition is to be used when drug causality is one of other possible causes for the described clinical event. Information on drug withdrawal may be lacking or unclear.

The essential distinctions between 'Probable' and 'Possible' are that in the latter case there may be another equally likely explanation for the event and/or there is no information or there is uncertainty with regard to what has happened after stopping.

In this criterion of unlikely, the clinical event, includes laboratory test abnormality and a temporal relationship to drug administration which makes a causal relationship improbable. This definition is intended to be used when the exclusion of drug causality of a clinical event seems most plausible. This provides plausible explanations of other drugs, chemicals or underlying disease being the causal factor to event.

Considering the next criterion *i.e.* Conditional/Unclassified, comprises clinical event, including laboratory test abnormality, reported as an adverse reaction, about which more data is essential for a proper assessment or the additional data are under examination. home.sweetim.com/?st=6&barid={DB5F5622-9E43-11E1-ABC8-E0699568B5E4}

Further Unassessable/Unclassifiable, it is a report suggesting an adverse reaction which cannot be judged because information is insufficient or contradictory, and which cannot be supplemented or verified.

The criteria that may render the connection 'Unlikely' are firstly the time relationship is improbable (with the knowledge at the time), and/or another explanation is more likely. The term 'Unclassified/ Conditional' is of a preliminary nature and is appropriate wher for a proper assessment, there is more data needed and such data are being sought, or are already under examination. Finally when the information in a report is incomplete or contradictory and cannot be complemented or verified, the verdict is 'Unclassifiable'. Since by far the most frequent categories in case reports are 'Possible' and 'Probable', the usual approach to using the system is to choose one of these categories (depending on the impression of the assessor) and to test if the various criteria fit with the content of the case report. If the report seems stronger one can go one step 'higher' (*e.g.* from 'Possible' to 'Probable'), if the evidence seems weaker one should try a 'lower' category. To see if that category is the right one or if it does again not seem to fit, the next adjacent term is tried. For drug-drug interactions the WHO-UMC system can be used by assessing the actor drug, which influences the kinetics or dynamics of the other drug (which has usually been taken over a longer period), in the medical context of the patient.

The four assessment criteria pertaining to causality evaluation are:

- The association in time and place between drug administration and event.
- Pharmacological information about the drug like associated side effects.
- Medical plausibility which would include characteristic signs and symptoms, laboratory tests and pathological findings.
- Likelihood or exclusion of other causes.

The significance of criteria may differ for different types of reactions, like for *e.g.* application site reactions, immunological reactions, immediate reactions, congenital malformations and cancer to name a few.

None of the available systems has been validated, *i.e.* that they consistently and reproducibly give a reasonable approximation of the truth. In this case validation would mean proving a procedure actually leads to the expected results. Although causality assessment is a very logical approach which has helped in approximate signal detection, there are some limitations of causality assessment which is ofcourse due to the events that are reported in a real life clinical situation and also individual to individual variation. This will also be more clear as we move forward to the chapter on special population. The support that causality assessment can render and cannot, is provided below also in a tabular form (Table 2) for better comprehension.

Table 2: The Dos' and Donts' of causality assessment

What causality assessment can do	*What causality assessment cannot do*
Decrease disagreement between assessors	Give accurate quantitative measurement of relationship likelihood
Classify relationship likelihood	Distinguish valid from invalid cases
Mark individual case reports	Prove the connection between drug and event
Improvement of scientific evaluation; educational	Quantify the contribution of a drug to the development of an adverse event
	Change uncertainty into certainty

The do's about causality assessment:

- Can decrease the disagreement between assessors
- Can classify relationship likelihood which is semi-quantitative analysis.
- Can educate and improve scientific assessment.

The dont's about causality assessment:

- Cannot give the exact quantitative measurement of relationship likelihood.
- Cannot distinguish valid from invalid cases.
- Cannot prove the connection between drug and event
- Cannot quantify the contribution of a drug to the development of an adverse event.
- Cannot change the uncertainity into certainity.

Table 3: Summary of terms related to causality assessment

Term	*Description*	*Comment*
Certain	A clinical event, including laboratory test abnormality, occurring in a plausible time relationship to drug administration and which cannot be explained by concurrent disease or other drugs or chemicals. The	It is recognized that this stringent definition will lead to very few reports meeting the criteria, but this is useful because of the special value of such reports. It is considered

Table 3: (*Contd...*)

Table 3: (*Contd...*)

Term	*Description*	*Comment*
	response to withdrawal of the drug (dechallenge) should be clinically plausible. The event must be definitive pharmacologically or phenomenologically, using a satisfactory rechallenge procedure if necessary.	that time relationships between drug administration and the onset and course of the adverse event are important in causality analysis. So also is the consideration of confounding features, but due weight must placed on the known pharmacological and other characteristics of the drug product being considered. Sometimes the clinical phenomena described will also be sufficiently specific to allow a confident causality assessment in the absence of confounding features and with appropriate time relationships, *e.g.* penicillin anaphylaxis.
Probable	A clinical event, including laboratory test abnormality, with a reasonable time sequence to administration of the drug, unlikely to be attributed to concurrent disease or other drugs or chemicals and which follows a clinically reasonable response on withdrawal (dechallenge). Rechallenge information is not required to fulfil this definition.	This definition has less stringent wording than for "certain" and does not necessitate prior knowledge of drug characteristics or clinical adverse reaction phenomena. As stated no rechallenge information is needed, but confounding drug administration underlying disease must be absent.
Possible	A clinical event, including laboratory test abnormality, with a reasonable time sequence to administration of the drug, but which could also be explained by concurrent disease or other drugs or chemicals. Information on drug withdrawal may be lacking or unclear.	This is the definition to be used when drug causality is one of other possible causes for the described clinical event.
Unlikely	A clinical event, including laboratory test abnormality, with a temporal relationship to drug administration which makes a causal relationship	This definition is intended to be used when the exclusion of drug causality of a clinical event seems most plausible.

Table 3: (*Contd...*)

Table 3: *(Contd...)*

Term	*Description*	*Comment*
	improbable, and in which other drugs, chemicals or underlying disease provide plausible explanations.	
Conditional/ Unclassified	A clinical event, including laboratory test abnormality, reported as an adverse reaction, about which more data is essential for a proper assessment or the additional data are under examination.	
Unassessible/ Unclassifiable	A report suggesting an adverse reaction which cannot be judged because information is insufficient or contradictory, and which cannot be supplemented or verified.	

5

Medical Dictionary for Regulatory Activities (MedDRA)

MedDRA's inception dates back to the 1990's when it was then known as ADROIT (Adverse Drug Reaction Online Information Tracking) post marketing safety database. As the name suggests in its abbreviated form *i.e.* MedDRA meaning Medicial Dictionary for (Medicines) Regulatory activities, it was planned for the usage in Pharmaceutical Industry especially for regulatory purposes confined to human medicines. It is a registered trademark belonging to the International Federation of Pharmaceutical Manufacturers Association which includes a neat and structured vocabulary of medical and other terminologies pertaining to human medicines. In 1993, the first version was called MEdDRA which meant Medicial Dictionary for (Medicines) Drug Regulatory affairs which was then renamed to MedDRA (Medicial Dictionary for (Medicines) Regulatory activities) by the International Conference on Harmonization (ICH) M1 Expert Working Group.

For accessing MedDRA, one would need to subscribe by paying to JMO or MSSO except for regulatory authorities for whom it is free of cost. The difference between dictionaries such as COSTART, HARTS, WHO-ART and MedDRA is that COSTART, HARTS, WHO-ART contain adverse reaction terms but MedDRA contains most of the terms from the adverse reaction terms from these dictionaries in addition to most of the terms from International Classification of Diseases (ICD9) and its clinical modification ICD9-CM. Although these terms from other dictionaries are present in MedDRA but they do not have the original relationships and hierarchical locations. Thus the motto of retaining these terms from other dictionaries in MedDRA was to facilitate the transfer of previously coded data in a particular database to a database using MedDRA. It was also for the intention of retaining the terms at data entry level, Lowest Level Term (LLT). Thus for instance, in WHOART, the preferred term (PT) cholesterol crystal emboli is located in the Platelet, bleeding and clotting disorders System Organ Class (SOC) whereas in MedDRA cholesterol crystal emboli is a LLT under PT Fat emboli located in the Injury, poisoning and procedural complications SOC.

MedDRA terminology consists of more than 60,000 terms, it contains terms for medical conditions, diagnoses, clinical signs, syndromes, laboratory and clinical investigations, symptoms including social circumstances, although it excludes certain items. The exclusion list of MedDRA is mentioned below, they are:

1. Does not provide definition of terms
2. Does not include demographic terms such as gender, age or race unless they are an element of medical condition
3. Does not include numerical expressions or measures of severity (no adjectives).
4. Animal Pharmacology, toxicology and veterinary terms are not included in MedDRA.
5. Does not include drug or device name unless it is representative of a medical diagnosis.

MedDRA comes as flat ASCII files and each of the MedDRA term is presented as words along with 8 numbered non logical code. MedDRA comes with a pack of several advantages and they are as listed below:

1. In recording baseline medical and social history and the names of clinical investigations during clinical studies.
2. To describe adverse events in Investigation Brochure (IB) or Development core safety information.
3. For electronic reporting of Suspected Unexpected Serious Adverse Drug Reactions to the clinical trial module of Eudravigilance regulatory safety database in The European Union.

4. In Recording and reporting adverse events during clinical studies.
5. In summary tables of adverse events to be included in the registration dossier for new product as recommeneded by the ICH E4M guideline on the Common Technical Document.
6. To present adverse reactions in the Company Core Safety Information and in the reference safety information, like the package insert and Summary of Product Characteistics (SPC) for marketed medicines.
7. For recording and expedited reporting of adverse reactions for marketed products as per regulations in EU, Japan, US, Canada and Australia.
8. For coding in individual case safety reports. MedDRA finds it use in coding of the following fields: medical history of disease and surgical procedures, past drug history: indications and reactions, adverse reaction or event, therapeutic indication for suspect drug, effects of rechallenge, cause of death.
9. In line listings and summary event tabulations for Periodic Safety Update Reports (PSURs).
10. MedDRA is multiaxial, which means that a Preferred Term (PT) with its Lowest level terms (LLTs) are presented in more than one SOC.

What does MedDRA include?

The terms in MedDRA are arranged in 5 hierarchical levels (as provided in Fig. 1). The levels are listed below:

1. Lowest level term or LLT
2. Preferred term or PT
3. High level terms or HLT
4. High level group terms or HLGT
5. System Organ Class or SOC
6. Lowest level terms are in the order of 60,000 in number. Similar LLTs are linked to the same PT which of the order of 16,000 in number. PTs associated with similar medical conditions are in turn grouped under some 1600 HLTs. HLTs are grouped under some 300 or more HLGTs. HLGTs are clustered under 26 SOCs

(provided in Table 1). This is represented as a figure below. Lowest level terms are at the bottom of the hierarchy and are large in number. This is to ensure that when an individual or HCP reports an adverse reaction, the same or very similar term analogous to the reported term (verbatim) is found in MedDRA as a LLT. Also there are some LLTs which are "non- current" and such LLTs must be used only for conversion of historical coded data and not the current data.

Number	***Level of terms***
26	SYSTEM ORGAN CLASS
332	HIGH LEVEL GROUP TERMS
1683	HIGH LEVEL TERMS
16751	PREFERRED TERMS
62348	LOWEST LEVEL TERMS

Fig. 1: MedDRA structure based on Hierarchy from top to Botttom

For the purpose of data presentation MedDRA allocates one SOC as primary location to a preferred term and 4 SOC locations for a given preferred term as secondary location. Seondary locations of SOCs are important since they may aid in finding all cases relevant to a medical condition. Some databases where MedDRA is not utilized to fullest potential may not be able to find secondary locations.

Table 1: The system organ class which includes 26 terms is as listed below

1. Blood and lymphatic system disorders
2. Cardiac disorders
3. Congenital, familial and genetic disorders
4. Ear and labyrinth disorders
5. Endocrine disorders
6. Eye disorders
7. Gastrointestinal disorders
8. General disorders and administration site conditions
9. Hepatobiliary disorders
10. Immune system disorders
11. Infections and infestations
12. Injury, poisoning and procedural complications
13. Investigations
14. Metabolism and nutrition disorders
15. Musculoskeletal and connective tissue disorders
16. Neoplasms benign, malignant and unspecified (incl cysts and polyps)
17. Nervous system disorders
18. Pregnancy, puerperium and perinatal conditions
19. Psychiatric disorders
20. Renal and urinary disorders
21. Reproductive system and breast disorders
22. Respiratory, thoracic and mediastinal disorders
23. Skin and subcutaneous tissue disorders
24. Social circumstances
25. Surgical and medical procedures
26. Vascular disorders

Search in MedDRA:

The verbatim or as reported term is matched with a LLT in MedDRA. Further there are browsers which start searches with SOCs and then getting to an appropriate LLT enroute HLGTs, HLTs and PTs. Also sometimes the narratives are scanned for coding of appropriate terms. It has to be remembered that when there are adverse events along with diagnosis and symptoms plus signs, then only diagnosis can be coded.

Coding signs and symptoms is optional in such a case. But if there are any signs and symptoms which are not a part of diagnosis, then both needs to be coded.

Data analysis and presentation of an adverse event that has been coded using MedDRA is a little complex due to a large number of terms, the best suitable levels and groupings for a specific purpose and multiaxiality. This could be best explained by considering a case of a parallel group clinical trial involving 100 patients in each treatment arm C and D respectively. If adverse events were coded using legacy dictionary such as COSTART, we may see an adverse event such as paraesthesia occurring in 7% patients in Treatment arm C and 9% patients in Treatment arm D. But in case of adverse event coding using MedDRA, the differences are stark because of specific grouping. However if more specific symptoms of paraesthesia would have been reported the differences in treatment arms would be much lesser. This may thus dilute the differences between the 2 treatment arms. This is because PTs are more specific for a reported verbatim or adverse event. However if we go higher up in hierarchy using MedDRA, like say HLTs for paraesthesia *i.e.* paraesthesia and dysesthesias, the proportion of 7 and 9% in respective treatment groups would remain same even using MedDRA. But if there is an investigational finding like HLT WBC analysis, this would fall under the Investigations SOC and can be quite complex. For WBC analysis HLT, the PTs would be WBC increased, WBC decreased, WBC count normal, WBC count abnormal. This would be rather difficult in comparison of effects between 2 treatment groups for WBC analysis. In some other instances, albeit there might not be any contradictory terms for a specific analysis but may be medically very different to the extent that the same HLT may be represented for a serious or a more milder or benign form of the disorder in question.

Rules that govern MedDRA:

1. Abbreviations which are not vague, are LLTs and are unpunctuated are allowed in MedDRA.
2. British English is referred in PTs and American English for LLTs.
3. While anatomical location of terms under primary and secondary SOCs, pathological process takes precedence over anatomical location.

Eg: PT nervous system disease congenital has its primary location in SOC: congenital, familial and genetic disorders and secondary location in nervous system disorders SOC

4. Reports of an investigational finding and reports of an apparent medical condition is differentiated in MedDRA. *i.e.* Investigational finding would go into the Investigations SOC and a medical condition would go into the anatomical location SOC.
5. In MedDRA, a PT is associated with only one HLT and HLGT of a given SOC unlike a PT finding representation in more than one SOCs *i.e.* primary and secondary locations respectively.

MedDRA finds its use as the largest, multiaxial, hierarchical dictionary not only in coding adverse reactions but also in recording clinical safety data. With better understanding of this sophisticated software, complexities can be unravelled and newer benefits can be assessed like signal detection with regards to new adverse reactions of marketed medications as well as evaluating clinical safety data of relatively newer drugs.

6

Signal Detection

Pharmacovigilance predominantly involves the identification and evaluation of safety signals. Signal refers to a concern about an excess of adverse events compared to what would be expected to be associated with a product's use. Information that is reported on a possible causal relationship between an adverse event and a drug, the relationship being unknown or incompletely documented previously is a signal. It should be an early information and credible at the same time. Further investigations are generally essential to confirm if the product at all caused the event. It is possible that even a single well documented case report can be viewed as a signal, particularly if the report describes a positive re-challenge or if the event is extremely rare in the absence of drug use. Usually more than a single report is required to generate a signal, depending upon the seriousness of the event and the quality of information. After a signal is identified, it should be further assessed to determine whether it represents a potential safety risk and whether other action needs to be taken. Post-marketing data and other sources, such as preclinical data and events associated with other products in the same pharmacologic class can give rise to signals.

However a neat and meticulous analysis of the benefit- risk of the drug should also be done alongside. The benefit risk evaluation report should consider the following features:

INTRODUCTION

- Brief description of the drug and where marketed.
- Indications for use, by country if there are differences.
- Alternative therapies, including surgery.
- Very brief description of the major safety problem.

A brief introduction must consist of a brief summary of the drug along with a mention of the countries where the product is marketed. A country wise listing of the Indications for which the drug is used needs to be stated, if the indications vary according to countries. Alternative therapies including surgery must also be mentioned. A very brief description regarding the major safety problem must also be included in the introductory part.

BENEFIT EVALUATION

- Epidemiology and natural history of the target disease(s).
- Purpose of treatment (*e.g.* cure, prophylaxis).
- Summary of efficacy and general toleration data compared with other treatments or no treatment.

The Benefit evaluation should comprise of the epidemiology and natural history of the targeted disease. Further the treatment aspect which would include the use of the drug either for cure or prophylaxis should be included also. The efficacy summary of the drug must entail the tolerance of the product used with a comparator study of other treatments. This summary must also highlight the quality of life, compliance of therapy, outcomes of the therapy.

RISK EVALUATION

- Introduction.
- Weight of evidence for the suspected risk.
- 3 Detailed presentations and analyses of data on the new suspected risk.
- Probable and possible explanations.

- Preventability, predictability and reversibility of the new risk.
- The issue as it relates to alternative therapies and no therapy.
- Review of the complete safety profile of the drug, using diagrammatic representations when possible ('risk profiles'); when appropriate focus on, for example, the three most common and the three most medically serious ADRs.
- Provide similar profiles for alternative drugs.
- When possible, estimate the excess incidence of any adverse reactions known to be common to the alternatives.
- When there are significant adverse reactions that are not common to the drugs compared, highlight important differences between the drugs.

Thus as it is discussed above the risk evaluation contains a description of the suspected risk associated with the drug. The extent to which the evidence related to the drug related risks is supported needs to be further highlighted. Also analysis and possible explanations related to the risk associated with the drug should be included. Next a diagrammatic representation of the safety-risk profile needs to be depicted which would give clarity on the safety and associated risks pertaining to a drug. The diagrammatic representation should project three most common and three most serious ADRs related to a drug. Also the more commonly occurring ADRs need to be compared to the alternative drugs being used. Further the ADRs which are not common to other alternative drugs used must be highlighted and the differential analysis must be done.

BENEFIT–RISK EVALUATION

- Summarise the benefits as related to the seriousness of the target disease and the purpose and effectiveness of treatment.
- Summarise the dominant risks (seriousness/severity, duration, incidence).
- Summarise the benefit–risk relationship, quantitatively and diagrammatically if possible, taking into account the alternative therapies or no treatment.
- Provide a summary assessment and conclusion.

Here the whole benefit and risk assessment is taken into consideration. The benefit-risk related to the therapy at hand is summarized herein. Quantitative evaluation is necessary because the ratio can thus be arrive at.

OPTIONS ANALYSIS

- List all appropriate options for action.
- Describe the pros and cons and likely consequences (impact analysis) of each option under consideration, taking alternative therapies into account.
- If relevant, outline plans or suggestions for a study that could provide timely and important additional information.
- If feasible, indicate the quality and quantity of any future evidence which would signal the need for a re-evaluation of the benefit–risk relationship.
- Suggest how the consequences of the recommended action should be monitored and assessed.

  After the benefit-risk is analysed thoroughly, the option analysis is done which details regarding various action steps that needs to be taken, especially when risk outweighs benefits. Also an account on the way the action plan needs to be monitored is taken into consideration.

Lack of assimilation among diverse information sources, such as prescription event monitoring databases, spontaneous reporting databases, linked administrative databases and medical records obstructs early detection of adverse reactions. Consequently many pharmaco-vigilance methods have visible dodges and in such a scenario, pharmaceutical firms need to proactively identify and expeditiously manage emerging safety risks. Thus to capitalize on the best accessible information from plethora of data sources, prospective signals needs to be detected in earlier stages of product development via processes which make use of sophisticated tools and programs.

When different doctors independently report the same unknown and unexpected adverse drug experiences with a particular drug, this can be considered as an important signal. Signals may consist of only a few cases and an important signal may not be statistically prominent. Signal testing and explanation require further study and many of them remain unconfirmed due to scientific limitations or lack of funding.

At various stages of risk identification and assessment, systematic examination of the reported adverse events by using statistical or mathematical tools, or so-called data mining, can provide additional information about the existence of an excess of adverse events reported for a product.

UNDERSTANDING DATA MINING

Data mining is an analytic process designed to explore data in search of consistent patterns and/or systematic relationships between variables and then validate the findings by applying the detected patterns to new subsets of data. The ultimate goal of data mining is prediction and predictive data mining is the most common type of data mining.

There are three stages in data mining:

- ***Initial exploration:*** This stage usually starts with data preparation which may involve cleaning data, data transformations, selecting subsets of records and in case of data sets with large numbers of variables, performing some preliminary feature selection operations to bring the number of variables to a manageable range. Then depending on the nature of the problem, this first stage of the process of data mining may involve anywhere between a simple choice of straight forward predictors for a regression model, to elaborate exploratory analysis using a wide variety of graphical and statistical methods in order to identify the most relevant variables and determine the complexity and general nature of models that can be taken into account in the next stage.
- ***Model building or pattern identification with validation/ verification:*** This stage involves considering various models and choosing the best one based on their predictive performance, *i.e.* explaining the variability in question and producing stable results across samples. There are variety of techniques developed to achieve this goal, many of which are based on the so called competitive evaluation of models, *i.e.* applying different models

to the same data set and then comparing their performance to choose the best.

- Deployment, *i.e.* the application of the model to new data in order to generate predictions: This final stage includes using the model selected as best in the previous stage and applying it to new data in order to generate predictions or estimates of the expected outcome.

Data mining to aid in signal detection has been used in post marketing surveillance studies, but not in clinical trial studies. Using these tools during clinical trials would reduce time in the interchange between researchers, clinicians and statisticians and thus allow clinical researchers to do close-to-real-time data analysis. But data mining alone are insufficient for signal detection and other processes such as collection, delivery of adverse events, triaging of potential signals, and chalking out pharmacovigilance plans are equally vital. Early detection of signals during clinical trials can avoid fiscal damages to the organization as well save a lot of time and efforts.

By applying data mining techniques to large adverse event databases, such as FDA's AERS or VAERS, it may be possible to identify unusual or unexpected product-event combinations warranting further investigation. Data mining can be used to boost existing signal detection strategies and is especially useful for assessing patterns, time trends, and events associated with drug-drug interactions. Data mining is not a tool for establishing causal attributions between products and adverse events. The methods of data mining currently in use usually generate a score comparing (1) the fraction of all reports for a particular event (*e.g.*, heart failure) for a specific drug (*i.e.*, the "observed reporting fraction") with (2) the fraction of reports for the same particular event for all drugs (*i.e.*,"the expected reporting fraction"). This analysis can be refined by adjusting for aspects of reporting (*e.g.*, the reporting year) or characteristics of the patient (*e.g.*, age or gender) that might influence the amount of reporting. Data mining can be limited to an analysis for drugs of a specific class or for drugs that are used to treat a particular disease. The score generated by data mining quantifies the disproportionality between the observed and expected values for a given product-event combination and is compared to a threshold that is chosen by the analyst. If the score exceeds the specified threshold then it leads to a potential excess of adverse events. When applying data mining to large databases (such as AERS), it is not unusual for a product to have several product-event combinations with scores above a specified threshold. The lower the threshold defined, the greater the likelihood that more combinations will exceed the threshold, and will warrant further investigation. Several data mining methods have been described and may be worth considering, such as the Multi-Item Gamma Poisson Shrinker (MGPS) algorithm, the Proportional Reporting Ratio (PRR) method and the Neural Network approach. Although all of these approaches are inherently exploratory or hypothesis generating, they may provide insights into the patterns of adverse events reported for a given product relative to other products in the same class or to all other products. Caution needs to be exercised when making such comparisons, because voluntary adverse event reporting systems such as AERS or VAERS are subject to a variety of reporting biases, like some instances could reflect concomitant treatment, not the product itself, and other factors, including the disease being treated, other comorbidities or unrecorded confounders, may cause the events to be reported. Submission of incomplete or duplicate reports, underreporting, or reporting stimulated by publicity or litigation may be additional alarms with regard to AERS or VAERS. If data mining results are submitted to FDA, they should be presented in the larger appropriate clinical epidemiological context. This should include:

1. A description of the database used
2. A description of the data mining tool used (*e.g.*, statistical algorithm, and the drugs, events and stratifications selected for the analyses) or an appropriate reference
3. A careful assessment of individual case reports and any other relevant safety information related to the particular drug event combination of interest (*e.g.*, results from preclinical, clinical, pharmacoepidemiologic, or other available studies).

Data mining algorithm called the Multi-item gamma poisson shrinker (MGPS) is used to interrogate spontaneous reporting database because of its ability to see the drug-drug interactions. In this case, the ratio of an observed adverse drug event to the total number of adverse events around millions, is obtained to detect a signal using Bayesian statistical analysis.

Some of the data mining techniques include the following:

Predictive modeling is a technique used to develop a model to relate a dependent variable with a set of independent variables in a manner similar to multiple regression analysis. There are two types of predictive modeling: classification, for categorical dependent variables, and value prediction, for continuous dependent variables. Classification is appropriate if the goal is to predict group membership of new records based on their characteristics (independent variables). Using classification, the most influential variable is identified and used to split the data into groups. This is then repeated with the next most influential variable until the data are fully characterized. The core of predictive data mining include: boosting, stacking and meta learning.

Clustering or Database Segmentation

Clustering uses an algorithm that segregates a database by evaluating the dissimilarity between records. Pairs of records are compared by the values of the individual fields within them, and clustering into groups provides fast and effective ordering in large datasets. Segmentation could be used to group patients with similar symptoms or diagnoses to determine whether there is a drug association. Thus, clustering is a technique of choice if the goal is to reduce a large sample of records to a smaller set of specific homogeneous subgroups (clusters) without losing much information about the whole sample. Because of the heterogeneity among clusters, this analysis can also be helpful in hypothesis development about the nature of the variation between subgroups.

Link Analysis

Link analysis refers to methods that identify associations or links between records or sets of data. It assesses associations by using an 'if x then y' type rule, by assessing patterns of behavior or by identifying similar time sequences of events.

Deviation Detection

Deviation detection looks for outliers or values that deviate from the norm and can be seen either graphically or statistically. Visualization techniques—such as scatter plots or histograms, multidimensional graphs for multivariate data, and time series plots—are used to determine patterns hidden in data. Statistical methods are then employed to measure the significance of deviations once they have been detected. This process could be used to identify patients with idiosyncratic reactions or unusual symptoms that could be related to medication and may constitute an adverse drug event signal.

Other techniques use Safety Data Mining (SDM)/disproportionality methods to identify adverse events that are reported with greater than expected frequency (statistical independence). Frequency is assessed against the background of all other drugs and events, and results are used for hypothesis generation. Another statistical tool is the Bayesian methodology to estimate relative reporting rates (risks) of adverse events. It is a tool for further analysis of potential signals and detection of complex dependencies in the data.

Automated signal detection methods which are used these days cannot replace clinical reviewers but can assist with difficult task of screening huge numbers of drug-adverse events for potential signals. Here evaluation for a significant occurrence of disproportionalities or dependencies between drug-event pairs is done which are based on an underlying model of statistical association. Currently detection algorithms based on Bayesian analysis for signal generation is being used by the WHO and FDA. This method has a good overall sensitivity as against low specificity. This could be attributed to certain limitations such as, small number of occurrences of each drug-event association in database and the fact that semantic information existing in controlled vocabularies used to code adverse events (like MedDRA, WHO-ART, COSTART, ICD etc) in case reports is not taken into account.

There is a continual urge for newer strategies to proactively identify and expeditiously control emerging risks in today's zero-tolerance ambience. Hence while understanding that the most advanced set of tools are required for developing a thorough and well-understood safety profile, there is a need to establish an optimal signal-to-noise ratio. For this, there needs to be a balance found between the sensitivity, specificity and false negative and false positive signals. This is essential because, a larger quantum of false positive signals may indirectly prevent patients from getting effective treatment. Likewise a larger chunk of false negative signals may lead to potential adverse drug reactions being missed. Also, many drug-drug interactions are possible to be detected only after the drug has hit the market. This could be a major threat to the geriatric population, since they are subject to administration of a lot of concomitant drugs. This will be discussed in detail in the subsequent chapter.

Signal detection is usually done considering the following points:

- ***Hypothesis generation:*** By selecting a possibly relevant association
- ***Signal strengthening:*** Preliminary assessment of the available evidence
- Signal follow up

DATA OF A SIGNAL COMPONENTS

- Qualitative which includes the clinical information.
- Quantitative which includes the epidemiological information.
- Experimental
- Develops over time

Criteria for selecting a signal:

- Unknown adverse reaction and not known or labeled one
- Unexpected reaction
- Expected but unlabelled
- Strong statistical connection and not a weak link.
- Low background frequency
- Specific and characteristic and not unspecific and trivial
- An objective event and not subjective
- Typically drug related event or critical term and not a common disorder type.
- Serious event
- High potential relevance

A signal is likely to be relevant in case if the below mentioned conditions arise:

- In case of early warning indicated by new adverse reaction and new drug.

- In case of an important drug being widely used for a serious indication
- When serious reactions are accounted.
- Large number of cases and rapid reporting happens.
- Regulatory intervention for prevention of the conditions being reported.
- When there is a change in benefit/risk ratio
- For scientific and educational value.

FDA believes that the methods described above will permit a sponsor to identify and preliminarily characterize a safety signal. The actual risk to patients cannot be known from these data because it is not possible to characterize all events definitively and because there is invariably under-reporting of some extent and incomplete information about duration of therapy, numbers treated, etc. Safety signals that may warrant further investigation may include, but are not limited to, the following:

1. New unlabeled adverse events, especially if serious;
2. An apparent increase in the severity of a labeled event;
3. Occurrence of serious events thought to be extremely rare in the general population;
4. New product-product, product-device, product-food, or product-dietary supplement interactions;
5. Identification of a previously unrecognized at-risk population (*e.g.*, populations with specific racial or genetic predispositions or co-morbidities);
6. Confusion about a product's name, labeling, packaging, or use;
7. Concerns arising from the way a product is used (*e.g.*, adverse events seen at higher than labeled doses or in populations not recommended for treatment);
8. Concerns arising from potential inadequacies of a currently implemented risk minimization action plan (*e.g.*, reports of serious adverse events that appear to reflect failure of a RiskMAP goal)
9. Other concerns identified by the sponsor or FDA: Even after 45 years of experience in the area of drug safety since the thalidomide tragedy, there are still many safety issues that arise and a highly

regulated pharmaceutical industry is incessantly compelled to withdraw licensed medicines for drug safety reasons. The crux is that, there is still a continued toxicity associated with modern day drugs. Why are the loopholes and lacuna pertaining to drug delivery still persistent?

The reasons are:

1. ***Quantum of patients:*** The number of patients representing a clinical trial of new drug licensing applications in the United Kingdom is only just over 1500. Albeit for new chemical entities, the rising regulatory demands for supplementary information before approval have presumably increased the average numbers of patients in applications but nevertheless, the numbers remain too undersized to detect uncommon or rare adverse drug reactions (ADRs), even if these are serious. Thus, because of this problem associated with numbers of patients being enrolled for clinical trials and also the inclusion/exclusion criteria, drug safety depends very largely on the supervision of medicines once they have been marketed.
2. Next reason, is that the type of patients who receive licensed medicines in real life clinical situation are very different from the kinds of volunteers and patients who are enrolled into pre-marketing clinical trials. The patients in formal clinical trials almost always have only one disease being treated with one drug. The drug, once licensed, is likely to be used in various other populations for whom the drug is not tested because such patients are not enrolled then during clinical trials like for instance geriatric or the elderly population. These patients seem to have more than one disease and be treated by more than one drug *i.e* polypharmacy. The drug may also be used in paediatric patients, who are generally excluded from initial clinical trials. The formal clinical trials may be a better test of efficacy than they are of safety under the practical conditions of everyday clinical usage.
3. Yet another problem is that doctors may be slow or ineffective in detecting and reporting adverse drug effects. Also in some cases the reactions may occur on long term/prolonged usage or chronic use and still some cases the reactions may take time to elicit it effects because of a lapse period.

4. Another reason is that many drugs that are withdrawn from the market are due to infrequent and very rare adverse effects. Thus expecting them to be shown up during the very short duration clinical trials and in limited set of population is little too unrealistic. Thus we need to gear up to have a sound and effective tool in place for monitoring total post-marketing safety experience.

   The large comprehensive databases such as the General Practice Research Database (GPRD) will hopefully change the situation in the future and will be more widely used for signal detection and evaluation. These databases record, in quite huge and representative populations, all usage of many specific medicines and clinical outcomes and can be used to methodically screen for and evaluate serious adverse events. Because they contain all-inclusive and ample information on some important information, such as age, sex, dose and clinical events on all patients in the represented population, they are systematic compared with spontaneous reporting systems. They may offer a better likelihood of detecting long-latency adverse reactions, effects on growth and development and other such forms of adverse experience.

Some of the difficulties due to numbers, patient populations and so on were recognized quite early. Now we shall give some interesting observatios as pointed out by the Committee on Safety of Drugs in the United Kingdom. The Committee on Safety of Drugs in the United Kingdom said – quite astonishingly – in its last report (for 1969 and 1970) that 'no drug which is pharmacologically effective is without hazard. Furthermore, not all hazards can be known before a drug is marketed'. Prescribers notion that licensed drugs are 'safe' proves wrong when a very small proportion of licensed drugs have to be withdrawn because of unexpected drug toxicity. Moreover patients themselves may have high expectations that licensed drugs are 'completely safe' rather than having a safety profile that is acceptably safe in the context of the expected benefit and nature of the underlying health condition. The Committee on Safety of Medicines, the successor in the United Kingdom to the Dunlop Committee, investigating this and related problems, recognized a Working Party on Adverse Reactions. This group, under the chairmanship of Professor David Grahame-Smith, published its second report in July 1985. The report supported the continuation of methods of spontaneous reporting by professionals but at the same time suggested that post-marketing surveillance (PMS) studies should be undertaken on newly marketed drugs intended for widespread long-term use'; the report also mentioned record linkage methods and prescription-based methods of drug safety surveillance as representing areas of possible progress. Similar reviews and conclusions have emerged from the United States since the mid-1970s. A series of events in the United States recently created a renaissance of curiosity in drug safety evaluation and management. Additional resources at the Food and Drug Administration (FDA) for drug reviews through user fees and established target timelines for FDA reviews was provided by the Prescription Drug User Fee Act (PDUFA) of 1992. The shorter approval times lead to some medications being approved sooner in the United States than that in Europe in contrast to the pre-PDUFA experience. But then, it was seen that a few highly visible drug withdrawals led to a perception that perhaps drugs were being approved too quickly. A published meta-analysis estimated that 106 000 fatal adverse reactions occurred in the United States in 1994. This and other articles stimulated considerable public, congressional and regulatory attention on plummeting the societal encumberance of drug reactions and medication errors. As a result, greater awareness, thought and resources are currently being devoted to signal generation and evaluation by the FDA, industry and academic centres. Moreover, efforts are in progress to develop better tools to administer recognized risks through a multiplicity of interventions, such as communications with healthcare providers and patients, restricted product distribution systems and other mechanisms. Further efforts are being focused on measuring the success of these risk management interventions. This new initiative represents a elementary shift in the safety model in the United States and offers new challenges to pharmacovigilance professionals. In fact, the shift is not restricted to the United States as both the FDA and the EMEA in 2005 issued guidance documents for industry on signal detection, evaluation, good pharmacovigilance practice and recommendations for managing risks after the approval. It is now a well accepted fact that the safety of drug depends not only on drug licensing by regulatory bodies but also on post-marketing drug safety surveillance, pharmacovigilance. It is also important to note that the same post-marketing information needed to confirm new safety signals is also needed to refute signals and protect the ability of patients to benefit from needed medicines that may be under notion or doubt due to spurious signals.

Table 1: Drug withdrawn from market due to ADRs

Drugs withdrawn in the United Kingdom by the marketing authorization holder or suspended or revoked by the Licensing Authority

Brand name (drug substance)	***Year action taken***	***Major safety concerns***
Secholex (polidexide)	1975	Safety concerns because of impurities
Eraldin (practolol)	1975	Oculomucocutaneous syndrome
Opren (benoxaprofen)	1982	Hepatotoxicity, serious skin reactions
Devryl (clomacran phosphate)	1982	Hepatotoxicity
Flosint (indoprofen)	1982	Gastrointestinal toxicity
Zomax (zomepirac)	1983	Anaphylaxis
Osmosin (indomethacin-modified release)	1983	Small intestine perforations
Zelmid (zimeldine)	1983	Neurotoxicity
Flenac (fenclofenac)	1984	Lyell's syndrome
Methrazone (feprazone)	1984	Serious skin reactions, multi-system toxicity
Althesin (alphaxolone plus alphadolone)	1984	Anaphylaxis
Pexid (perhexilene)	1985	Hepatotoxicity, neurotoxicity
Suprol (suprofen)	1986	Nephrotoxicity
Merital (nomifensine)	1986	Haemolytic anaemia
Unicard (dilevalol)	1990	Hepatotoxicity
Glauline eye drops 0.6% (metipranolol)	1990	Uveitis
Halcion (triazolam)	1991	Psychiatric reactions
Micturin (terodiline)	1991	Arrhythmias
Teflox (temafloxacin)	1992	Multi-system toxicity
Centoxin (nebacumab)	1993	Mortality
Roxiam (remoxipride)	1994	Aplastic anaemia
Volital (pemolin)	1997	Hepatotoxicity
Romazin (troglitazone)	1997	Hepatotoxicity
Serdolect (sertindole)	1998	Arrhythmias
Tasmar (tolcapone)	1998	Hepatotoxicity
Ponderax (fenfluramine)	1998	Cardiac valvular disease
Adifax (dexfenfluramine)	1998	Cardiac valvular disease

Table 1: *(Contd...)*

Table 1: *(Contd...)*

Brand name (drug substance)	***Year action taken***	***Major safety concerns***
Posicor (mibefradil)	1998	Drug interactions
Trovan (trovafloxacin)	1999	Hepatotoxicity
Grepafloxacin (Raxar)	1999	QT interval prolongation
Prepulsid (cisapide)	2000	QT interval prolongation
Alec (pumactant)	2000	Adverse comparative trial results
Droleptan (droperidol)	2001	Increased cardiac risks
Lipobay (cerivastatin)	2001	Rhabdomyolysis
Kava-Kava	2001	Liver toxicity
Anorectic agents (amfepramone, phentermine)	2000	Heart valve disorders
Vioxx (rofecoxib)	2004	Increased cardiovascular event risks
Non-proprietary (co-proxamol)	2005	Use in suicide
Bextra (valdecoxib)	2005	Steven-Johnson syndrome

CASE STUDIES RELATED TO DRUG WITHDRAWAL FROM MARKET: (ALSO PROVIDED AS TABLE 1 ABOVE)

1. ***Diethylstilbestrol:*** Diethylstilbestrol (DES) was used since 1941 for four different indications gonnorheal vaginitis, atrophic vaginitis, menopausal symptoms and post partum lactation suppression to prevent breast engorgement. This drug was also used off-label to prevent adverse pregnancy outcomes in case of women with history of miscarriage. However a link between DES and vaginal clear cell adenocarcinoma was published in the New England journal of medicine. Prevention of miscarriage as an indication was further removed by FDA and added pregnancy as a contraindication during DES usage. In the year 1975, 25 and 100 mg tablets of DES were ordered for withdrawal from the market.
2. ***Phenformin:*** Anti-diabetic drug phenformin from the biguanide class, was withdrawn from the market due to high risk of lactic acidosis, claimed to be fatal in 50% of the cases. The formal proceedings which began in mid 1977 by FDA led to an eventual withdrawal in the year 1978.

3. ***Ticrynafen:*** This uricosuric diuretic drug was used for uric acid lowering action, formerly marketed as an antihypertensive. This was withdrawn from the market in 1982 owing to a number of instances of serious hepatic injury.
4. ***Zimelidine:*** A selective serotonin uptake inhibitor, Zimelidine was the first of its kind to be marketed to treat depression. This drug has been banned worldwide due to fatal incidences of peripheral and/or central neuropathy known as Guillain barre syndrome. Further there were also cases of hypersensitivity reaction including skin exanthema, flu like symptoms, arthralgias and sometimes eosinophilia reported which led to the drug withdrawal from the market.
5. ***Phenacetin:*** Phenacetin in the form of A.P.C. or Aspirin-Phenacetin-Caffeine was used as an analgesic. However in the year 1983, US FDA ordered the withdrawal of drugs containing phenacetin, since it resulted in carcinogenic and kidney damaging effects. There were numerous reports which depicted urothelial neoplasms especially urothelial carcinoma of the renal pelvis due to phenacetin administration.
6. ***Methaqualone:*** In 1984, addiction and overdose resulted in the withdrawal of this product.
7. ***Nomifensine:*** Nomifensine, an antidepressant, is chemically a tetrahydroisoquinoline. This antidepressant was registered in 98 countries and was first introduced in Germany in the year 1976 and in the United Kingdom in the year 1977. Being a New chemical entity (NCE), it was chemically different from any other antidepressant. The mode of action of Nomifensine was the inhibition of presynaptic reuptake of biogenic amines in the brain thus helping increasing the concentration of the amines. Besides it also helped in the inhibition of reuptake of dopamine and Nomifensine's metabolite supported the inhibition of reuptake of serotonin with less pronounced effects on noradrenaline. Thus by increasing concentrations of amines it helped in the treatment of depression. Since it did not have overdose adverse effects such as cardiotoxicity and epileptogenic activity, it was found to be a suitable alternative to those subgroups of patients who had cardiovascular diseases or epilepsy and for patients suffering from parkinson's disease due to its dopaminergic properties.

Nomifensine proved to be a boon then in 1980s when, tricyclic antidepressants caused deaths due to poisoning at a proportion second to barbiturates. Tricyclic antidepressants and monoamine oxidase inhibitors were associated with many adverse reactions and thus nomifensine became a drug of choice in treating depression since it was also exceptionally well tolerated in an instance of overdose.

But unfortunately in the period between 1978 and 1979, there were 4 reported cases of females (aged 25–64) suffering from hemolytic anaemia. Like wise between 1981 and 1982, there were 3 more cases of haemolytic anaemia. But since there was an occurrence of the adverse event only in 1 out of 150 000 patients, no regulatory action was initiated. Symptoms of chronic haemolytic anaemia included lethargy, fatigue and breathlessness. And the acute haemolytic anaemia patients showed signs of backache, loin pain, jaundice, haematuria and in certain cases fever, renal failure and cardiorespiratory collapse. Another diagnosis which confirms hemolytic anaemia is the Coombs' (anti-globulin) test being positive. Coombs' test being positive was observed in all the four patients. Also it was observed that on dechallenge *i.e.* withdrawal of medication nomifensine, the patient made full recovery (outcome was full recovery). Haemolytic anaemia is a condition wherein, the antibodies to the drug or its metabolites attack the blood cells. There is a destruction of blood cell, which is due to the combining of antigen on cell surface with the antibody. Anaemia thus results from cell damage. Severe haemolysis can result in prerenal uraemia and renal failure.

But there was no cause-effect relationship between the drug and adverse event (*i.e.* between nomifensine and haemolytic anaemia) despite of many retrospective and prospective immunological studies being conducted. In these studies it was determined that some patients with positive Coombs' test did not have haemolysis, on the other hand some showing negative Coombs' test suffered blood dyscrasia, haemolytic anaemia. Thus Coombs' test was not a marker for judging the adverse event. But in 1981 in UK, there were supportable evidence of the causal relationship between nomifensine and haemolytic anaemia *i.e* a suspected link was established and hence haemolytic anaemia was added on as side effect in the 1981 data sheet. This spurred in further immunological investigations which suggested an immunological basis for haemolytic anaemias. Also further studies in 19 patients proved the antibody response to one or more metabolites of nomifensine and ex vivo antigens rather than nomifensine itself. This indicated specificity for unidentified early or late metabolite. Only 5 out of 19 were reactive to nomifensin.

From 1983 onwards the number of reports increased from 5 in 1983, 12 in 1984 and 18 including 3 fatalities in 1985 in UK. Between Jan 1983 and mid june 1985, there were 1 in 20,000 reports of haemolytic anaemia. But the number of reports increased from 1 in 20,000 to 1 in 4000 between mid june and end of November 1985. WHO defines a rare incidence as an adverse event which occurs at a level above 1 in 10,000 wherein benefits no longer outweighs the risks. Thus it was concluded that benefits of nomifensine did not outweigh the risk of haemolytic anaemia. The adverse event was further reported in 4 more patients in the year 1986, out of which one patient died and this led to the withdrawal of the drug from worldwide markets because of the risk of haemolytic anemia. Also there were some deaths which were linked to immuno-haemolytic anemia.

8. ***Triazolam:*** A benzodiazepine was used a sedative to treat severe insomnia. In 1991, the drug was withdrawn from the UK market due to psychiatric adverse reactions. But in the US it still continues to be marketed.
9. ***Terodiline:*** Terodiline was first marketed in a relatively small market of Scandinavia in the year 1965 as an anti-anginal agent. During its use as an antianginal agent, urinary retention an anticholinergic property of the drug proved to be an adverse drug reaction. Thus the drug was re-developed for another clinical use in the early 1980s for urinary incontinence due to detrusor instability. But in the year 1991, due to prolonged QT interval, the drug was withdrawn from the market. It is important to note that drugs that prolong QT interval are considered more likely to cause torse de pointes. Thus QT interval prolongation has been considered as a marker to differentiate safer drugs from drugs that are relatively less safer which belong to the same class.

Thus one significant thing that needs to be done during drug development of drugs belonging to the same class here is a retrospective analysis pertaining to safety issues of other drugs belonging to the same therapeutic, pharmacological, chemical class. Thus an analysis pursuant to the withdrawal of prenylamine and lidoflazine could have avoided a lot of bitter experiences related to terodiline.

A list of drugs such as Prenylamine in 1988, lidoflazine in 1989 and terodiline in 1991 were withdrawn from the market due to QT liability. And similar was the reason to anticipate withdrawal of other drugs such as Terfenadine, astemizole, cisapride, sertindole, grepafloxacin, droperidol, thioridazine, levacetylmethadol. Certainly Terodiline withdrwal from the market was an important turning point in the pharmacovigilance arena. The potent secondary pharmacological effect such as potent anticholinergic side effect of Terodiline which was seen as adverse drug reactions actually directed redevelopment from clinical point of view for alltogether different set of indications. The adverse effect of Terodiline was on cardiac repolarization and QT interval prolongation on the surface Electrocardiogram (ECG).

From a regulatory perspective, should terodiline been approved considering its pro-arrhythmic potential? Well yes, because at the time of approval of Terodiline in 1986, there was no other drug available for treatment of urinary incontinence with comparable efficacy and risk-benefit ratio. The main adverse anticholinergic reactions reported were rather mild in nature and hence the benefits outweighed the risk. But in the year 1991, due to reported adverse reactions of QT interval prolongation, the drug was withdrawn from the market since also the risk outweighed the benefits shown by the drug. It was replaced by the drug oxybutynin in the year 1991. Hence regulatory bodies while approving drugs, are unwilling to approve drugs that prolong QT interval and more ready to approve drugs without a QT liability. Also it has to be kept in mind, that in certain cases even if the drug shows a prolonged QT interval but if they show an acceptable risk-benefit profile the drug may be approved. Ziprasidone or arsenic trioxide is a classic example of such approval due to acceptable risk-benefit profile.

10. ***Temafloxacin:*** A fluoroquinolone antibiotic, was used to treat lower respiratory tract infections, genital and urinary infections. Due to severe adverse reactions including allergic reactions and hemolytic anemia, the drug was withdrawn from the market in 1992. These adverse reactions also led to three deaths.
11. ***Flosequinan:*** A quinolone vasodilator, which has direct relaxing effects on peripheral arteries and veins, was used in the treatment of congestive heart failure. Marketed as Manoplax®, the product was withdrawn from the market due to several hospitalizations and deaths.
12. ***Alpidem:*** Alpidem used as an antianxiety drug, caused serious hepatotoxicity, and the product was withdrawn from most of the markets in the year 1996. This drug never received FDA approval. It was withdrawn from the French market in 1994.
13. ***Chlormezanone:*** An anxiolytic and muscle relaxant, chlormezanone was withdrawn from many markets in 1996 due to serious toxic epidermal necrolysis reports.
14. ***Fenfluramine:*** Fenfluramine, a drug used as an antiobesity medication was introduced in the US market in 1973. The drug was withdrawn from the US market in 1997 because of reports related to heart valve diseases, pulmonary hypertension and cardiac fibrosis. After which it was also withdrawn from other markets.
15. ***Tolrestat:*** Tolrestat is an aldose reductase inhibitor, used in the treatment of diabetes. Alredase (Tolrestat) was withdrawn in 1997 after the appearance of severe liver toxicity and deaths among several patients.
16. ***Terfenadine:*** An antihistamine, marketed under the brand name seldane in US entered market in 1985 for the treatment of allergic rhinitis. But in 1990, FDA issued reports regarding risk factors associated with concomitant use of the drug with macrolide antibiotics and ketoconazole due to evidences of ventricular arrythmias in consumers. In 1997, FDA recommended that Seldane be withdrawn from the market.
17. ***Mibefradil:*** Posicor, brand name for mibefradil was used for the treatment of hypertension and chronic angina pectoris. Dangerous interactions with other drugs led Mibefradil's withdrawal.

Posicor, a novel antihypertensive blocks both the T-type and L-type calcium channels, with greater selectivity for the T-type. It did not induce reflex tachycardia but slightly reduced the heart rate. Posicor reduced the activity of certain liver enzymes that are important in helping the body eliminate many other drugs. Posicor inhibited cytochrome P450 2D6 and 3A4 and could interact by increasing the plasma concentrations of concomitantly administered drugs. This led to the increased accumulation of drugs which reached dangerous levels in the body. Interactions, particularly with those drugs that also affect liver metabolism, appeared to cause catabolism of important abdominal muscles in a few people. The interaction was considered extremely dangerous. The withdrawal came after reports of dangerous and even fatal interactions with at least 25 other drugs, including common antibiotics, antihistamines, and cancer drugs. Posicor, which went onto the general market in August 1997 was consumed by almost 200000 Americans and nearly double that number worldwide for both hypertension and angina. Its withdrawal was a logistical nightmare for many large cardiology practices faced with the need to notify patients that they would need to obtain a different prescription.

18. ***Tolcapone:*** Tasmar, a brand name for Tolcapone is used for the treatment of Parkinson's disease. Eventually, in 1998 Tasmar was withdrawn from the market due to reports of occurences of hepatotoxicity.
19. ***Temazepam:*** Sold under the trade names Restoril, Euhypnos, Normison, Remestan, Tenox and Norkotral. Diversion, abuse and a relatively high rate of overdose deaths resulted in the withdrawal of this product from Norway and Sweden markets. It still continues to be available under strict purview in other markets including US.
20. ***Astemizole:*** An H1 receptor antagonist shows its effects as anticholinergic and antipruritic. In 1999, Hismanal trade name for Astemizole was found to cause Arrhythmias and prolonged QT interval due to interactions with other drugs and thereby resulted in this product's withdrawal.
21. ***Grepafloxacin:*** A quinoline anti-bacterial agent to treat bacterial infections was marketed under the brand name Raxar. Prolonged

QT interval led to cardiac events and sudden death were reasons attributed to the withdrawal of this product.

22. ***Troglitazone:*** Rezulin, a brand name for troglitazone was used for lowering and controlling blood sugar levels in case of patients with type II diabetes. Since 1997, increasing number of patients developed serious liver toxicity on consumption of this drug. The authorities requested to withdraw this product from market.
23. ***Alosetron:*** In 2000, Lotronex associated risk of fatal complications of constipation resulted in the withdrawal of this product in 2000, but was reintroduced on a restricted basis in the year 2002.
24. ***Cisapride:*** A gastroprokinetic agent, acted directly as serotonin 5-HT5 receptor agonist and indirectly as parasympathomimetic for increasing motility in the upper gastrointestinal tract. Cisapride, a prescription drug treatment was approved for severe nighttime heartburn experienced by adult patients with gastroesophageal reflux disease (GERD) that does not adequately respond to other therapies. The year 1999, reported 341 reports of heart rhythm abnormalities including 80 reports of deaths which were associated with use of cisapride. Most of these adverse events occurred in patients who were taking other medications or suffering from underlying conditions known to increase risk of cardiac arrhythmia associated with cisapride. Cisapride was marketed under the brand names prepulsid and propulsid. Cisapride was withdrawn in many countries due to risk of cardiac arrhythmias in the year 2000.
25. ***Amineptine:*** Referred by tradenames Survector, Maneon, Directim, Neolior, Provector and Viaspera, Amineptine is used as an atypical antidepressant.

    In 2000, Survector. Hepato-toxicity, abuse potential and dermatological side effects were reasons for withdrawal of this product.
26. ***Phenylpropanolamine:*** In 2000, Propagest, Dexatrim. High doses of this drug, *i.e* 75 mg twice daily taken by women under 50 years for weight loss, was seen to cause stroke. Thus this product was withdrawn due to this fatal side effect.
27. ***Trovafloxacin:*** Trovafloxacin, a trifluoronaphthyridone derivative is used as fluoroquinolone antimicrobial drugs. It is a

broad spectrum antibiotic that inhibits the uncoiling of supercoiled DNA in various bacteria by blocking the activity of DNA gyrase and topoisomerase IV. As a class, the most common adverse effects involve the CNS and gastrointestinal tract. Liver enzyme abnormalities have been noted in 2%–3% of patients, and liver toxicity is reported infrequently. Since the authorization of this drug marketed under the brand name Trovan, in the United States in December 1997, 152 cases of serious hepatic events due to trovafloxacin were reported to the US Food and Drug Administration (140 cases) and to the European Agency for the Evaluation of Medicinal Products (12 cases as of July 1998). Because the frequency of serious adverse reactions to trovafloxacin was well out of proportion to that seen in other drugs in this class, the manufacturer withdrew trovafloxacin from the European markets. The drug remains available in the United States for very restricted indications.

28. ***Cerivastatin:*** Cerivastatin was first approved as a lipid-regulating agent in 1997. Was known under brand names Baycol and Lipobay and withdrawn in the year 2001. By 2000 a total of 549 cases of rhabdomyolysis associated with cerivastatin use had been reported. Consequently a signal was issued regarding an association between cerivastatin, myopathy and rhabdomyolysis. Thus, the prescribing information was changed to include a contraindication for the combined use of cerivastatin and gemfibrozil, another lipid-regulating medicine. A similar action was taken and a warning issued to alert prescribers to the possibility of rhabdomyolysis occurring with all statins. A regulatory action was taken to contraindicate the combined use of cerivastatin and gemfibrozil. The manufacturer voluntarily withdrew cerivastatin from the market on the grounds of an increased risk of rhabdomyolysis, particularly when used in combination with gemfibrozil.

FDA today announced that Bayer Pharmaceutical Division is voluntarily withdrawing Baycol (cerivastatin) from the U.S. market because of reports of sometimes fatal rhabdomyolysis, a severe muscle adverse reaction from this cholesterol-lowering (lipid-lowering) product. The FDA agrees with and supports this decision. Baycol also known as Cerivastatin, which was initially approved in the U.S. in 1997, is a member of a class of cholesterol lowering drugs that are commonly referred to as "statins." Statins lower cholesterol levels by blocking a specific enzyme in the body that is involved in the synthesis of cholesterol. While all statins have been associated with very rare reports of rhabdomyolysis, cases of fatal rhabdomyolysis in association with the use of Baycol have been reported significantly more frequently than for other approved statins. Fatal rhabdomyolysis reports with Baycol have been reported most frequently when used at higher doses, when used in elderly patients, and particularly, when used in combination with gemfibrozil (LOPID and generics), another lipid lowering drug. FDA has received reports of 31 U.S. deaths due to severe rhabdomyolysis associated with use of Baycol, 12 of which involved concomitant gemfibrozil use. Rhabdomyolysis is a condition that results in muscle cell breakdown and release of the contents of muscle cells into the bloodstream. Symptoms of rhabdomyolysis include muscle pain, weakness, tenderness, malaise, fever, dark urine, nausea, and vomiting. The pain may involve specific groups of muscles or may be generalized throughout the body. Most frequently the involved muscle groups are the calves and lower back; however, some patients report no symptoms of muscle injury. In rare cases the muscle injury is so severe that patients develop renal failure and other organ failure, which can be fatal. Bayer Pharmaceutical Division has announced plans to withdraw Baycol to the pharmacy level. Pharmacies will be instructed to return the product to the manufacturer for a refund. Patients who are taking Baycol should consult with their physicians about switching to alternate medications to control their cholesterol levels. Patients taking Baycol who are experiencing muscle pain or are also taking gemfibrozil should discontinue Baycol immediately and consult their physician. There are five other statins available in the U.S. that may be considered as alternatives to Baycol. They are: lovastatin (Mevacor), pravastatin (Pravachol), simvastatin (Zocor), fluvastatin (Lescol), and atorvastatin (Lipitor).

When crises arise, whether they are real or suspected, regulatory authorities are expected to meet them efficiently. The regulatory authority has powers to suspend registration, impose special conditions, or severely restrict use to certain patients or prescribers. The authority may require manufacturers to change the product information in a specified manner. These decisions are normally communicated by drug alerts, general letters to doctors and pharmacists, press statements, through websites, newsletters and journal publications, depending on the type and urgency of the message and those who are being addressed. Many national authorities have identified the need for developing an organizational plan for managing risks and for communication and action during crises. Regulators themselves often react under duress in a drug safety crisis within a legislative or administrative framework that is inadequate or excessively restrictive. There should be clear yet flexible operating procedures so that their response is not delayed, unnecessarily complicated, or unduly cautious (undue caution may result in removal of a product from the market even when there may be no justification and a more thoughtful and less drastic response would be appropriate). The pharmaceutical industry has prime responsibility for the safety of medicines, from the start of drug development and thereafter throughout the lifetime of the drug. Many companies have developed innovative and efficient monitoring systems that have contributed to the detection of new safety signals. Encouraged by the 1998 Erice Declaration on Communicating Drug Safety, communication and exchange of information between the industry, regulatory authorities and the public has improved, which has more recently been further supported by the establishment of the community database (Eudravigilance Database) in December 2001, in London.

29. ***Rapacuronium:*** Rapacuronium, marketed under the tradename Raplon® a rapidly acting, non-depolarizing neuromuscular blocker formerly used in modern anaesthesia. As a depolarizing agent it did not cause initial stimulation of muscles before weakening them. From 19 months after its approval, on 27 March 2001, was voluntarily withdrawn by the manufacturer. The Raplon® package insert leaflet had listed bronchospasm as an adverse event in 3.2% patients in premarketing clinical trials. It was observed however that there were several serious adverse bronchospasm events along with some unexplainable fatalities. But the causality was unknown in each of the cases, due to multiple drug administration and associated concomitant conditions. It was also seen that although the event formed a part of labeling, but the severity of events including mortality were not seen as a part of clinical trials.

30. ***Rofecoxib:*** Marketed under the brand name Vioxx, Ceoxx and Ceeoxx, Rofecoxib is a Non-Steroidal anti-inflammatory (NSAID) drug for the treatment of osteoarthritis, acute pain and dysmennorhoea. It was approved by the FDA in the year 1999 and was withdrawn from the market in the year 2004. This was a voluntary withdrawal from the market due to concerns such as increased risk of heart attack and stroke which was linked to a long term usage and high dosage. There were around 88,000 to 140,000 cases of serious heart disease reported. Myocardial infarction was the reason behind this drug's withdrawal from the market.

    The adverse cardiovascular outcomes were due to vasoconstriction, platelet aggregation and vascular proliferation. This is because Rofecoxib being a selective COX-2 inhibition causes thromboxanes' activity to dominate the prostacyclins activity. It was also indicated at the time of approval in the pharmacological studies of celecoxib and rofecoxib, that the selective COX-2 (present in endothelium) inhibitory activity would actually result in no production of prostacyclin, thereby showing no platelet aggregation, no vasodilatation, and no prevention of vascular proliferation. Also since COX-2 inhibitors does not affect COX-1 found in platelets, thromboxane produced by COX-1 takes over prostacyclin resulting in adverse cardiovascular events.

31. ***Coproxamol:*** Is a paracetamol/dextropropoxyphene combination product indicated for the relief of mild to moderate pain marketed under the brand names distalgesic, cosalgesic and dolgesic. This product was associated with upto 400 accidental or intentional fatal overdoses every year till its withdrawal. Since the drug's benefits did not outweigh the risks associated, the drug was withdrawn from clinical use.

32. ***Hydromorphone extended release:*** Marketed under brand names Palladone and Dilaudid is a very potent centrally acting analgesic drug. Hydromorphone was withdrawn from the market in the year 2005, because of the risk for potentially fatal adverse effects when given with alcohol concomitantly. Administration with alcohol disrupts the formulation's extended release mechanism, thereby causing rapid hydromorphone release and achieving peak concentrations of 2-16 fold compared to, when there is a drug intake with water.

33. ***Thioridazine:*** The generics of the antipsychotic drug were discontinued in Canada in the year 2005 due to lack of convincing safety information. This was due to the associated prolonged QT intervals resulting in potentially fatal cardiac arrhythmia including sudden death and torsade de pointes. There were three reported deaths between 2000 and 2005. Albeit the innovator preparation (Novartis' Mellaril) was voluntarily withdrawn from Canadian market in 2001, other generic products continued in the market then.
34. ***Pemoline:*** Pemoline, marketed under the brand name Cylert®, is a second line therapy for patients with attention deficit hyperactivity disorder. This product was withdrawn from US market in 2005 because of hepatotoxicity. Thirteen cases of acute liver failure have been reported to FDA since Cylert's marketing in 1975. The rate of reporting ranges 4–17 times the rate expected in the general population. The long latency between initiation of Cylert® administration and occurrence of liver toxicity leading to limiting the recognition of association coupled with under reporting may be attributable factors to a lower estimate of the cases reported. The earlierst onset of hepatic abnormalities occurred 6 months after the initiation of Cylert®. It led to severe liver damage leading to death and liver transplant within four weeks of onset of signs and symptoms of liver failure.
35. ***Natalizumab:*** Natalizumab: Natalizumab, a humanized monoclonal antibody is used against the cellular adhesion molecule α4-integrin. It is co-marketed by Biogen-Idec and Elan as Tysabri and was previously named as Antegren. The ability of inflammatory immune cells to attach to and pass through the cell layers lining the intestines and blood-brain barrier is reduced by Natalizumab.Based on a one year short-term data,the Food and Drug Administration (FDA) approved Natalizumab in December 2004. However, three months later, the drug was withdrawn because of reports that two patients on the Natalizumab-plus-beta inferon group developed progressive multifocal leukoencephalopathy (PML), a brain disease caused by a virus. This occurred when the drug was administered concomitantly with interferon beta-1a, an immunosuppressive drug used in multiple

sclerosis treatment. One of the patients died as a result and the other developed severe neurological disabilities. Further, a clinical trial patient who had received Natalizumab infusions for the treatment of Crohn's disease developed a fatal case of PML. These three patients were among approximately 3,000 patients receiving Natalizumab. In February 2005 Natalizumab was withdrawn from the market pending safety review and agreement on a risk reduction program with the FDA. In March 2006, after a review of safety information the FDA Central Nervous System Committee voted to approve reintroduction of the drug for first-line therapy for relapsing-remitting multiple sclerosis (MS) under a special prescription program. As of October 2009, 24 cases of PML had been reported since its reintroduction and by Jan 2010, there were 31 cases attributed to Natalizumab, depicting a sharp increase in the number of fatalities.

36. ***Ximelagatran:*** Ximelagatran, marketed as Exanta/Exarta was an anticoagulant introduced to replace warfarin therapy. Astrazeneca had submitted an application for marketing authorization to the EMEA for the indications, *viz.*: prevention of stroke and other thromboembolic complications associated with atrial fibrillation (irregular heartbeat with ineffective contraction of the upper chambers of the heart. In 2006, Astrazeneca announced the withdrawal of the pending applications of the product from the market due to liver toxicity reports associated with the product and discontinue distribution to countries where the drug was approved. It was notified to the European medicines agency (EMEA) by Astrazeneca to withdraw an application for centralized marketing authorization for Ximelagatran 36 mg film coated tablets. The voluntary withdrawal was due to an adverse event report of severe liver injury during long term treatment of 11 days and abnormal hepatic laboratory values during short term treatment.

37. ***Pergolide:*** Pergolide, marketed under the trade name Permax, an ergoline based dopamine receptor agonist was used for the treatment of Parkinsons disease. Pergolide, having similar effects to Dopamine was used in Parkinson's disease where the neurotransmitter levels of Dopamine are low. Pergolide belongs

to a class of medications called dopamine agonists and is used with levodopa and carbidopa to manage the symptoms (tremors and slowness of movement) of Parkinson's disease. Permax was approved in 1988 for Eli Lilly and Company as an adjunctive therapy with levodopa in Parkinson's disease. Valvular heart disease was first described in association with pergolide in 2002. Also there were some reports in New England Journal of Medicine studies confirming findings associating pergolide with increased chance of regurgitation (backflow of blood) of the mitral, tricuspid, and aortic valves of the heart. Valve regurgitation is a condition in which valves don't close tightly, allowing blood to flow backward across the valve. Symptoms include shortness of breath, fatigue and heart palpitations. In 2003, FDA asked Lilly to add valvulopathy (abnormality of cardiac valves) to the warnings section of Permax labeling, at which time a Dear Healthcare Practitioner letter was sent by Lilly. In 2006, the warning was upgraded to a black box warning, the FDA's strongest form of warning, because of new data concerning risks of heart valve damage. Owing to risk of serious damage to patients' heart valves, manufacturers of pergolide took the decision of voluntarily removing the drugs from the market. Not only were the innovator product of Pergolide marketed by Valeant Pharmaceuticals withdrawn, but also the two generic versions of pergolide manufactured by Par and Teva withdrawn.

38. ***Tegaserod:*** Tegaserod sold under the name Zelnorm® increases the action of a chemical called serotonin in the intestines, which speedens the movement of stools through the bowels. It is used to treat severe, chronic, irritable bowel syndrome (IBS) in women who have constipation (and not diarrhoea) as their main bowel problem and is used to treat chronic constipation in patients younger than 55 years old. Tegaserod is not for use in people with diarrhea as the main symptom of their irritable bowel condition. An analysis of data collected on over 18,000 patients demonstrated adverse cardiovascular events in 13 of 11,614 patients treated with Zelnorm as compared with 1 of 7,031 patients treated with placebo (a rate of 0.01%). In the year 2007, the U.S. FDA requested that Novartis withdraw Zelnorm from the market. A causal relation between prescriptions of the drug and increased risks of heart attack or stroke was the observation done by FDA.

39. ***Aprotinin:*** Aprotinin, marketed under the brand name Trasylol, is used in the prevention of blood loss and to reduce the need for blood transfusion in patients undergoing cardiopulmonary bypass during coronary artery bypass graft surgery (CABG). Aprotinin is an inhibitor of fibrinolysis and is isolated from bovine lung tissue. It was first approved in the U.S. in 1993 for patients at high risk for bleeding during surgery, but in 1998 the use was widened for the use during cardiopulmonary bypass. In the year 2007 Bayer Pharmaceutical Co. was requested to suspend the marketing of aprotinin (Trasylol) by the U.S. Food and Drug Administration (FDA). This was due to the fact that the drug increased risks of death and stroke. It was published in The New England Journal of Medicine that the drug increased the risks of kidney failure, heart attack and stroke.
40. ***Lumiracoxib:*** Lumiracoxib is a non-steroidal anti-inflammatory drug (NSAID) that belongs to the group 'COX-2 inhibitors'. Marketed under the trade name Prexige®, it is used for symptomatic relief in the treatment of osteoarthritis of the hip and knee. In August 2007, Prexige was withdrawn from the market in Australia following 8 serious liver adverse events, including 2 deaths and 2 liver transplants. In the year 2007, the US Food and Drug Administration issued a not approvable letter for lumiracoxib, requiring additional safety data. The European Medicines Agency (EMEA) recommended the withdrawal of the marketing authorisations for all lumiracoxib-containing medicines, because of the risk of serious side effects affecting the liver. The EMEA's Committee for Medicinal Products for Human Use (CHMP) concluded that the risks of lumiracoxib-containing medicines are greater than their benefits. The CHMP therefore recommended that the marketing authorisation for these medicines should be withdrawn in all European Union (EU) Member States where they were approved.
41. ***Rimonabant:*** Rimonabant, marketed under the trade name Acomplia, was used as an anti-obesity drug. The drug was found to cause psychiatric side effects including suicidal tendencies. It has been banned in several countries including India. In the year 2008, the Drug Technical Advisory Board (DTAB) advised the government to withdraw the drug from the market.

42. ***Efalizumab:*** Efalizumab marketed under the trade name Raptiva® is used for the treatment of chronic moderate to severe plaque psoriasis. Efalizumab is an anti-CD11a antibody immunosuppressant drug. But due to the potential risk of patients developing progressive multifocal leukoencephalopathy (PML), the drug was withdrawn from the market. PML is a rapidly progressive infection of the central nervous system caused by the John Cunningham (JC) virus that leads to death or severe disability. But it was also observed that the risk of an individual patient developing PML is rare and is generally associated with long-term use. Usually, PML occurs in people whose immune systems have been severely weakened and often leads to an irreversible decline in neurologic function and death. The labeling for efalizumab was updated on October 16, 2008, to warn of the risk for life-threatening infections, including PML. Consequently, after receiving reports of 4 patients with PML, 3 of whom died, the FDA issued a public health advisory. Due to the risk of PML, the European Medicines Agency and the FDA recommended suspension from the market in the European Union and the United States, respectively. In April 2009, Genentech Inc. announced a phased voluntary withdrawal of Raptiva from the U.S. market.
43. ***Sibutramine:*** An antiobesity drug, marketed under the a variety of brand names including Meridia, Reductil and Sibutrex was withdrawn from the market by Abbott laboratories in light of clinical trial data pointing to an increased risk for stroke and myocardial infarction. The study, called the Sibutramine Cardiovascular Outcomes Trial (SCOUT), demonstrated a 16% increase in the risk for serious cardiovascular events such as nonfatal heart attack, nonfatal stroke, the need for resuscitation after the heart stopped, and death in a cohort of patients given sibutramine compared with another given a placebo.
44. ***Gemtuzumab ozogamicin:*** Marketed by Wyeth under the trade name Mylotarg was a drug linked monoclonal antibody for the treatment of acute myelogenous leukemia. A black box warning was added to Gemtuzumab packaging in the first year of approval. There was an increased risk of Veno-Occlusive Disease (VOD) reported in the absence of bone marrow transplantation. But it was found later that VOD was observed, even following bone

marrow transplantation. The drug was withdrawn from the market in June 2010 due to drug increased mortality rates found in a clinical trial and also since the benefits did not outweigh the risks.

45. Rosiglitazone marketed under the brand name Avandia, is an antidiabetic drug. It functions as an insulin sensitizer by making the cells more responsive to insulin. The drug is associated with an increased risk of heart attacks. In Sep 2010, the European Medicines Agency recommended that the drug be suspended from the market. In Newzealand, the drug was withdrawn form market in April 2011.

The drug development programmes (DDP) need to gear up in characterizing relatively rare but potentially fatal clinical hazard. The drug development method fails to recognize problems associated with other members of the same chemical, pharmacological or therapeutic class of drugs. Thus a potential class related safety issue needs to be identified during the drug development process. Like for eg: QT interval prolongation is a concentration dependent Type A adverse reaction and which can be identified during the pre-clinical/clinical phase of the drug development. Which goes on to say further that the predictable events need to be recognised in the early stages of drug development.

The good news is that every stakeholder benefits. Manufacturers can enhance compliance with regulatory timelines, deliver superior quality data, cut down time spent in physician follow-up, increase brand protection with advance safety warnings, provide competitor product intelligence and potentially open new returns streams through product line extensions. Healthcare providers gain standard tools and processes for reporting adverse events that save time and offer a higher level of protection for their patients. Healthcare payers can make more informed coverage decisions with standardized data in hand. With standardization, regulators' safety reviews will be faster and defined. Ultimately, patients win with an efficient system that protects them, and, as a result, their perception of the industry will perk up.

7

Special Cases

Many studies have reported the huge impact that poor product quality, adverse drug reactions (ADRs), and medication errors have on health care in general and on patients' health in particular, but because most cases go undetected, estimating the actual scale of this burden is almost impossible. When people take medicines, they may suffer adverse clinical events, such as dizziness, headache, skin rashes, or other symptoms, but not all adverse events are caused by medicines; some may result from the patient's illness or condition, genetic or environmental factors, diet, or other causes. Adverse drug reactions are directly related to medicines and may result due to poor product quality, medication error (in prescribing, preparing, administering, or taking the medicine), or known/unknown pharmacological properties. There also cases where the product has no efficacy and hence does not elicit a said therapeutic effect as mentioned in the label or package insert leaflet. Also there are instances where the medication error, adulterated products, accidental administration which may lead to adverse drug reactions being fatal and life threatening in nature. Overdose, abuse of medicines, usage of medicines which are not approved, drug-drug interactions etc. also can lead to dangerous levels of drug concentration in blood and thereby result in adverse drug reactions. Thus cases also fall under the pharmacovigilance purview.

- Lack of efficacy reports

- Medication errors
- Accidental administration
- Substandard medicines
- Use of medicines for indications that are not approved and for which there are inadequate scientific basis.
- Abuse and misuse of medicines
- Adverse interactions of medicines with chemicals, other medicines and food.
- Overdose

Product quality: Monitoring the quality of products available in the marketplace should identify products that are defective, deteriorated, or adulterated because of poor manufacturing practices, inadequate distribution and storage, or tampering. Medicines that have lost their potency after being stored at high temperatures would fall under this category, for example, as would counterfeit products. Many studies have documented the circulation of counterfeit and substandard medicines.

Lack of efficacy: In this case the product that is administered by patients and result in adverse reactions is due to the lowered efficacy of the product. This means that the Active Pharmaceutical ingredient present in the product is not at a particular dose to produce a certain therapeutic effect. This may lead to an adverse reaction. Reports of lack of efficacy specifically for drugs used in the treatment of life-threatening conditions and for certain other medicinal products, such as contraceptives and vaccines, may represent a significant hazard, and in that sense may be a safety issue

Substandard medicines: Here the medicinal product is of substandard quality. This may be due to an adulteration by mixing spurious products or the Active Pharmaceutical Ingredient is a counterfeit substance. This ultimately results in adverse drug reaction.

Accidental administration: In the situation such as accidental administration, the patient consumes the product accidentally. This generally happens in case of children, when the product container is at accessible to children, and they consume the medication without consulting parents.

Accidental administration might lead to adverse reactions in the below mentioned set of conditions:

1. The product is a prescription product and is accidentally administered without prescription.
2. Is contraindicated in some instances *i.e* in a given situation, due to prevailing patient conditions, physician would not recommend prescribing.
3. *Has a warning of not to be consumed by children:* In this case the product is strictly not meant for children, but is consumed by a child.
4. *The dose exceeds a certain level:* In such a scenario, the product which even if accidentally administered is not harmful under normal doses but can do damage if the doses are high.

Medication errors: Medication error is defined as "any preventable event that may cause or lead to inappropriate medication use or patient harm while the medication is in the control of the health care professional, patient, or consumer".

Medication errors result from faulty systems, processes, and conditions that lead people to make mistakes or fail to prevent mistakes. Problems can result from illegible handwriting, use of dangerous abbreviations, overlooked interactions with other medicines, oral miscommunications, and sound-alike or look-alike products. In a nutshell medication errors may be caused due to errors in prescribing, drawing up and administration of the medication. The main focus of adverse events happening from such sort of a medication errors is the preventability. The processes need to be robust to avoid fatalities and ensure safety.

Use of medicines for indications that are not approved, and for which there are inadequate scientific basis: The approval of a product is imperative by the Drug authorities of a country *i.e* Food and Drug Administration. For every new indication the product is used for, there needs to be an approval from regulatory authorities. The authorities after meticulously scrutinizing the data regarding the product, sanctions a license for marketing. If the products are used without relevant approvals or there is no adequate scientific basis with regard the product, then there are all possibilities of an adverse drug reaction, to the extent which could be fatal and life threatening.

Abuse and misuse of medicines: The drug product in this case is wrongly used by the patient. In such instances the patient administers the drug even if it is not required for any health conditions. There might also be an excessive dose consumed by a patient which exceeds the maximum safe concentration and thus elicits toxic effects. Also certain drugs are contraindicated in certain prevailing conditions of a patient or to be used concomitantly along with other drugs that the patient consumes. Thus, if the patient administers a drug under such conditions then it may result in an adverse drug reaction.

Adverse interactions of medicines with chemicals, other medicines and food: When a particular medication is incompatible with a concomitant medication, a chemical or food consumed the output is an adverse interaction. In certain cases of a drug-drug interaction, the active ingredient of a medication interacts with a concomitant treatment medication which may result in a toxicity or sub therapeutic levels of the drug. Also there are examples of drug-food interaction, viz: antidepressants interact with tyramine containing food substances to produce hypertensive crisis.

Overdose: This is due to dose of a particular product being administered by the patient which is more than the actual dose. The drug levels thereby reach a level much higher than the maximum safe concentration. Due to this the adverse drug reaction is triggered in a patient.

Considering the scope of this book, we have touched at a preliminary level, the various other aspects of drug safety which could lead to adverse reactions. As seen, it is evident that all the types of special cases are due to the usage of medication in an unacceptable manner due to the lack of knowledge and information either on the part of the patient, health practitioner, pharmacist etc., or due to misuse of the product, or carelessness on part of the consumer etc. Lack of efficacy is an example of an ineffective drug, so here the drug is incapable of eliciting its desired efficacy. Substandard medicines are a example of adulteration of the formulation itself. Thus it can be seen that the chapter focuses on other than the conditions where the drug in itself is responsible for the adverse reaction. The details about these cases will be covered in subsequent editions of the book.

8

Special Population

When a new medicine is being developed, it goes through several phases of testing for safety and efficacy, first with animals, then with human volunteers. When a product is approved, however, it may have been tested in only a limited number of patients—orders of magnitude less than are likely to use the product once it is approved. Therefore, premarketing studies generate incomplete information on safety relative to the full profile of likely users, including sensitive groups whom clinical trials do not include, such as children, pregnant women, and the elderly. As a result, postmarketing surveillance is a critical tool for completing the safety and effectiveness profile of a new medicine.

The dose of a drug is a major determinant of its safety, and establishing a safe dose of a novel drug is a prime objective during clinical development. The design of pre-marketing clinical trials precludes the representation of important subpopulations such as children, the elderly and people with co-morbidities. Thus in such cases, the dose and dosage regimen which is safe and efficacious for these special groups of patients, viz: children, elderly, pregnant women and people with co-morbidities is not arrived at and fixed during clinical trials. Therefore, postmarketing surveillance (PMS) activities are required to monitor the safety profile of drugs in real clinical practice. Hence since the safety is monitored during real clinical practice, many safety issues surface up either because the dose doesn't match the individual requirements of those special population, or drug interactions occur due to the patients associated comorbidities etc. This particular chapter deals with the challenges due to which the clinical trials are often not conducted in such population prior to marketing. Thus, the safety of a drug is a major clinical consideration before and after it is marketed. Pharmacokinetic-pharmacodynamic modelling provides a method of predicting a clinically safe dose; consideration of drug pharmacokinetics in special populations may enhance safe therapeutics in a wider spectrum of patients.

Medications for the pediatric age group are rarely tested during clinical trials. A children specialist thus struggles to provide standard care to the pediatric lot since they have not been appropriately evaluated. Hence pediatrician prescribing medicines for children involves educated guesses about doses, safety and effectiveness. A lack of appreciation of the differences between children and adults often results in the inappropriate extrapolation of data derived from adults to the pediatric population. This situation is dangerous. The child is either deprived of the benefits of drug therapy because of lack of information or is exposed to unknown side effects. Thus, children under 2 years of age are affected by adverse reactions to medication and leads to critical injuries and death. It is very evident thus that additional drug testing in the pediatric population is imperative.

Below mentioned is a list of pediatric disasters:

1. Sulfanilamide elixir, an antibiotic, manufactured with solvent ethylene glycol, raspberry syrup as excipients caused renal failure which lead to deaths of many children.
2. Thalidomide, a sedative was safe for the mother but proved fatal to the fetus which led to severe limb abnormalities (phocomelia) in the fetus.
3. Chloramphenicol caused grey baby syndrome *i.e.* toxicity and deaths in children.

Thus formulations that suit the pediatric population with safe Absorption, Distribution, Metabolism and Excretion (ADME) properties, teratogenicity, appropriate dose for children population, dosing and safety issues associated with the product for children are very essential pointers to be considered while developing a product for children.

Some of the drugs which were marketed in the duration 2003–2005 set in alarm signals for the pediatric group. The pediatric advisory committee expressed safety concerns for these drugs requesting for an amendment in labeling:

1. Fentanyl transdermal patches were observed to have been misused leading to serious adverse outcomes including death.
2. The selective serotonin uptake inhibitors like sertraline and paroxetine led to neonatal withdrawal syndrome.
3. Following a controlled pediatric clinical trial, the causal relation between antidepressants such as nefazodone, citalopram, venlafaxine, sertraline with suicidality was confirmed.
4. Methylphenidate and amphetamines which were used to treat Attention Deficit Hyperactivity Disorder (ADHD) caused cardiovascular and psychiatric adverse events.

There are several reasons because of which a safety signal might not be identified till postmarketing in pediatric section, they are as enumerated below:

1. Relatively fewer number of pediatric population being recruited in atrial
2. Pediatric population recruited for phase 3 trials are based on information obtained in adults or little information obtained in the pediatric poplation. This is because very less number of children being included in a phase 1 pharmacokinetic and safety studies and phase 2 dose finding and safety studies.
3. The off label use of the products in pediatric population which are actually marketed for adults. Either the drug in question would have been studied in a particular subgroup and not in other subgroups for which they are used in a off label way or for the indication for which it is used it would not have been studied in any population subgroup at all.
4. The variations in dosing and dosing schedule that is observed in children across various age groups because of changes in the ADME patterns across such groups. This is further explained in detail below.
5. Breast milk exposures are not routinely evaluated for effects on the child.

6. Because of a deficit of formulations designed for pediatric use, many a times the formulation given for children are not tested for bioavailability, drug-drug, or drug food interactions, which might in turn lead to generation of adverse events.
7. Products which might be tested in a child during one stage of development for safety and efficacy may not apply in the other stages of the child's life.

Appropriately evaluated medicines should be given to the pediatric population to ensure safe and effective therapy. This requires the timely development of information on the proper use of medicinal products in pediatric patients of various ages and also the development of pediatric formulations of those products. Advances in formulation chemistry and in pediatric study design will help facilitate the development of medicinal products for pediatric use. Drug development programs needs to incorporate the pediatric patient population so as to obtain relevant and significant information including side effects, toxic doses, Maximum safe concentration and minimum effective concentration etc. This is very essential when a particular product is in future going to be used for children. However, this should be done without compromising the well-being of pediatric patients participating in clinical studies.

There are certain major hindrances due to which research in such populations has lagged behind than in adults. The major impediments for not involving special populations in clinical trials are as listed below:

1. ***Ethical:*** Since they are generally viewed by the medical research community as a vulnerable group that needs protection from the potential harm of participating in a drug study.
2. ***Technical:*** Technical difficulties, including the need for frequent blood sampling and the inability to measure endpoints such as pain and quality of life in very young children, have been cited as an impediment to testing drugs in children.
3. ***Logistics:*** Logistically, pediatric trials are often difficult to perform. For many pediatric diseases, such as infantile spasms and juvenile rheumatoid arthritis, a relatively small number of children are affected, so there are recruitment problems.

It is commonly perceived that drug use in children is infrequent and confined to a small number of drug classes, primarily antimicrobials, and that there is little financial incentive for industry to conduct major clinical trials of drug therapy in children. However, recent data indicate that increasing numbers of children in the United States are taking prescription medications. Ensuring the availability of evidence-based information on the efficacy, dosing and safety of medications commonly used in children not only is ethically appropriate but also seems a worthwhile economic investment for all the stake holders.

There are reasons why pediatric populations are more prone to adverse events from therapies and there may be reasons also why they go unrecognised. These are as listed below:

1. *Variations in disease process and / or drug disposition characteristics in different developmental stages of pediatric population:* As the child grows, several enzymatic, endocrinic, metabolic systems and processes are expressed for the first time, when the child is exposed to an infection or a specific condition and is subjected to a therapy. A disease manifestation is different for adults and children and so is the laboratory values; not only between an adult and child but also in the various stages of a child development. The different stages and age groups of the child are explained later in this chapter. Also the drug disposition characteristics (ADME) are different in various stages of drug development. Like for certain products the clearance of he drug product is cleared more rapidly in a older child than a younger one. Where as in other instances the product is clearance is more rapid in the younger as compared to the older child. This may lead to either overdosing or underdosing. Overdosing may precipitate adverse events and underdosing may not elicit the desired therapeutic effect and the condition may remain unresolved.
2. *Dificulties in determination of repercussions of drug exposure on child that have delayed effects as adverse events in later stage of their lives:* It is very difficult to assess in this case if the delay/ problem in growth, development or cognitive abilities of a child is due to the exposure to a particular drug therapy or were it to happen independent of any drug exposure. Like for instance, there might hav been a drug exposure in infancy or childhood which elicits the adverse events in the later part that is towards an adolescent age. Hence the adverse event goes unrecognised until the child turns

adolescent and at that point it is again difficult to say if there was a causal relation between the drug exposure and adverse event or was it an independent occurrence.

3. *Formulation issues with pediatrics:* Developing an apt formlation for the pediatric group is generally an issue to deal with. This is mainly because the excipients used alongside the active pharmaceutical ingredient may not be safe in children group as it may be for adults. Considering the cost-effectiveness part of the formulation, many sponsors are not keen on manufacturing pediatric formulations because of the heavy cost that is incurred on the same. It comes with a small profit margin. Generally acceptable formulations for pediatrics are liquid, but the smaller shelf life and risky solvents that accompany these formulations render them a major setback again. Compounded or extemporaneous preparations given to them often are not tested for bioavailability, drug-drug interactions or food-drug interactions. This leads to overdosing, underdosing or medication errors of the medication given to a child.
4. *Problems related to recognising and reporting of adverse events:* In this case the children many a times are not able to communicate the adverse events that they face to parents. Also the vice versa, parents will not be able to recognise the adverse events untill there are visible reactions such as vomiting, crying, breathing problems, diarrhoea etc. Also they might understand this for some mild changes related to food habits or growing process instead of an adverse event reaction and altogether ignore it.

Although they are generally viewed by the medical research community as a vulnerable group that needs protection from the potential harm of participating in a drug study as mentioned above. However, it can be argued that it is unethical to subject pediatric patients in clinical practice to the risks of therapy with medications that have not been adequately evaluated in their age group. Also as discussed earlier, there might be technical difficulties, including the need for frequent blood sampling and the inability to measure endpoints such as pain and quality of life in very young children, have been cited as an impediment to testing drugs in children. However, advances in clinical pharmacology such as population pharmacokinetics and sparse sampling (testing only a couple of samples from each child in a large group), along with increasing expertise in clinical epidemiology and outcomes research, are reducing these concerns. Improved tools for assessing pain and measuring quality of life are now available for use in younger groups. Likewise, logistically pediatric trials are often difficult to perform. For many pediatric diseases, such as infantile spasms and juvenile rheumatoid arthritis, a relatively small number of children are affected, so there are recruitment problems. But with increasing collaboration between researchers, the potential for multi-center trials will improve and facilitate the study of drug therapy, as has happened in pediatric oncology.

The decision to proceed with a pediatric development program for a medicinal product, and the nature of that program, involve consideration of many factors, including:

- The prevalence of the condition to be treated in the pediatric population
- The seriousness of the condition to be treated
- The availability and suitability of alternative treatments for the condition in the pediatric population, including the efficacy and the adverse event profile (including any unique pediatric safety issues) of those treatments
- Whether the medicinal product is novel or one of a class of compounds with known properties
- Whether there are unique pediatric indications for the medicinal product
- The need for the development of pediatric-specific endpoints
- The age ranges of pediatric patients likely to be treated with the medicinal product
- Unique pediatric (developmental) safety concerns with the medicinal product, including any nonclinical safety issues
- Potential need for pediatric formulation development

Of these factors, the most important is the presence of a serious or life-threatening disease for which the medicinal product represents a potentially important advance in therapy. This situation suggests relatively urgent and early initiation of pediatric studies. Any classification of the pediatric population into age categories is to some extent arbitrary, but a classification such as the one below provides a basis for thinking about study design in pediatric patients. Decisions on how to stratify studies and data by age need to take into consideration developmental biology and pharmacology. Thus, a flexible approach is necessary to ensure that studies reflect current knowledge of pediatric pharmacology. The identification of which age groups to study should be medicinal product-specific and justified. If the clearance pathways of a medicinal product are well established and the ontogeny of the pathways understood, age categories for pharmacokinetic evaluation might be chosen based on any "break point" where clearance is likely to change significantly. Sometimes, it may be more appropriate to collect data over broad age ranges and examine the effect of age as a continuous covariant. For efficacy, different endpoints may be established for pediatric patients of different ages, and the age groups might not correspond to the categories presented below. Dividing the pediatric population into many age groups might needlessly increase the number of patients required. In longer term studies, pediatric patients may move from one age category to another; the study design and statistical plans should prospectively take into account changing numbers of patients within a given age category.

The following is one possible categorization. There is, however, considerable overlap in developmental (*e.g.*, physical, cognitive, and psychosocial) issues across the age categories. Ages are defined in completed days, months, or years.

- Preterm newborn infants
- term newborn infants (0 to 27 days)
- infants and toddlers (28 days to 23 months)
- children (2 to 11 years)
- adolescents (12 to 16–18 years (dependent on region))

Preterm newborn infants: The study of medicinal products in preterm newborn infants presents special challenges because of the unique pathophysiology and responses to therapy in this population. The complexity of and ethical considerations involved in studying preterm newborn infants suggest the need for careful protocol development with expert input from neonatologists and neonatal pharmacologists. Only rarely will it be possible to extrapolate efficacy from studies in adults or even in older pediatric patients to the preterm newborn infant. The category of preterm newborn infants is not a homogeneous group of patients. A 25-week gestation, 500-gram (g) newborn is very different from a 30-week gestation newborn weighing 1,500 g. A distinction should also be made for low-birth-weight babies as to whether they are immature or growth retarded. Important features that should be considered for these patients include: (1) gestational age at birth and age after birth (adjusted age); (2) immaturity of renal and hepatic clearance mechanisms; (3) protein binding and displacement issues (particularly bilirubin); (4) penetration of medicinal products into the central nervous system (CNS); (5) unique neonatal disease states (*e.g.*, respiratory distress syndrome of the newborn, patent ductus arteriosus, primary pulmonary hypertension); (6) unique susceptibilities of the preterm newborn (*e.g.*, necrotizing enterocolitis, intraventricular hemorrhage, retinopathy of prematurity); (7) rapid and variable maturation of all physiologic and pharmacologic processes leading to different dosing regimens with chronic exposure; and (8) transdermal absorption of medicinal products and other chemicals. Study design issues that should be considered include: (1) weight and age (gestational and postnatal) stratification; (2) small blood volumes (a 500 g infant has 40 mL of blood); (3) small numbers of patients at a given center and differences in care among centers; and (4) difficulties in assessing outcomes.

Term newborn infants (0 to 27 days): While term newborn infants are developmentally more mature than preterm newborn infants, many of the physiologic and pharmacologic principles discussed above also apply to term infants. Volumes of distribution of medicinal products may be different from those in older pediatric patients because of different body water and fat content and high body-surface-area-to weight ratio. The blood-brain barrier is still not fully mature and medicinal products and endogenous substances (*e.g.*, bilirubin) may gain access to the CNS with resultant toxicity. Oral absorption of medicinal products may be less predictable than in older pediatric patients. Hepatic and renal clearance mechanisms are immature and rapidly changing; doses may need to be adjusted over the first weeks of life. Many examples of increased susceptibility to toxic effects of medicinal products result from limited clearance in these patients (*e.g.*, chloramphenicol grey baby syndrome). On the other hand, term newborn infants may be less susceptible to some types of adverse effects (*e.g.*, aminoglycoside nephrotoxicity) than are patients in older age groups.

Infants and toddlers (28 days to 23 months): This is a period of rapid CNS maturation, immune system development and total body growth. Oral absorption becomes more reliable. Hepatic and renal clearance pathways continue to mature rapidly. By 1 to 2 years of age, clearance of many drugs on a mg/kg basis may exceed adult values. The developmental pattern of maturation is dependent on specific pathways of clearance. There is often considerable inter-individual variability in maturation.

Children (2 to 11 years): Most pathways of drug clearance (hepatic and renal) are mature, with clearance often exceeding adult values. Changes in clearance of a drug may be dependent on maturation of specific metabolic pathways. Specific strategies should be addressed in protocols to ascertain any effects of the medicinal product on growth and development. Children achieve several important milestones of psychomotor development that could be adversely affected by CNS-active drugs. Entry into school and increased cognitive and motor skills may affect a child's ability to participate in some types of efficacy studies. Factors useful in measuring the effects of a medicinal product on children include skeletal growth, weight gain, school attendance, and school performance. Recruitment of patients should ensure adequate representation across the age range in this category, as it is important to ensure a sufficient number of younger patients for evaluation. Stratification by age within this category is often unnecessary, but it may be appropriate to stratify patients based on pharmacokinetic and/or efficacy endpoint considerations. The onset of puberty is highly variable and occurs earlier in girls, in whom normal onset of puberty may occur as early as 9 years of age. Puberty can affect the apparent activity of enzymes that metabolize drugs, and dose requirements for some medicinal products on a mg/kg basis may decrease dramatically (*e.g.*, theophylline). In some cases, it may be appropriate to specifically assess the effect of puberty on a medicinal product by studying pre- and post-pubertal pediatric patients. In other cases, it may be appropriate to record Tanner stages of pubertal development or obtain biological markers of puberty and examine data for any potential influence of pubertal changes.

Adolescents (12 to 16–18 years (dependent on region)): This is a period of sexual maturation; medicinal products may interfere with the actions of sex hormones and impede development. In certain studies, pregnancy testing and review of sexual activity and contraceptive use may be appropriate. This is also a period of rapid growth and continued neurocognitive development. Medicinal products and illnesses that delay or accelerate the onset of puberty can have a profound effect on the pubertal growth spurt and, by changing the pattern of growth, may affect final height. Evolving cognitive and emotional changes could potentially influence the outcome of clinical studies. Many diseases are also influenced by the hormonal changes around puberty (*e.g.*, increases in insulin resistance in diabetes mellitus, recurrence of seizures around menarche, changes in the frequency and severity of migraine attacks and asthma exacerbations). Hormonal changes may thus influence the results of clinical studies. Within this age group, adolescents are assuming responsibility for their own health and medication. Noncompliance is a special problem, particularly when medicinal products (for example, steroids) affect appearance. In clinical studies compliance checks are important. Recreational use of unprescribed drugs, alcohol and tobacco should be specifically considered. The upper age limit varies among regions. It may be possible to include older adolescents in adult studies, although issues of compliance may present problems. Given some of the unique challenges of adolescence, it may be appropriate to consider studying adolescent patients (whether they are to be included in adult or separate protocols) in centers knowledgeable and skilled in the care of this special population.

However the legislation passed by the US congress towards the end of 20th century, changed the scenario of pediatric drug development. The main elements of the legislations are listed below:

1. In response to the FDA issuance of a document known as the written request for pediatric studies, 6 months of additional marketing exclusivity for those products would be rendered. Renewed in 2002 in the Best Pharmaceuticals for Children Act (BPCA), this was first enacted in the Food and Drug administration Modernization Act (FDAMA) of 1997.
2. A final regulation was published by FDA in 1998 enacted as Pediatric Research Equity Act (PREA) of 2003, which mentions that if a sponsor who wishes to study a product in adults and would

like to use the same product in the pediatrics group needs to also conduct studies in children. With regards the same, the sponsor should submit a plan and timelines for the said studies.

3. If the manner in which a therapy behaves for a similar kind of disease in adults and children is the same, then the adult efficacy data can be extrapolated to the children group as well. But the dosing and safety studies in pediatric population are mandatory. This regulation was incorporated into the BPCA Act in the year 2002.
4. In accordance with the BPC Act, the results of the trials conducted in response to FDA's written request are posted in summary form on FDA's website. This is not the case with studies conducted in response to PREA.
5. In accordance with the BPCA, a specific product will be allocated 1 year special safety review after the additional 6 months exclusivity period. The adverse events should be intimated to the newly mandated office of pediatrics therapeutics after which a review needs to be presented to the Pediatrics Advisory Committee.

Under reporting is one major factor that we have seen in the population pool. This may be either due to lack of knowledge either by parents or care takers of the children concerned to interpret the observed pattern of events as an adverse reaction or the children not being able to recognise/communicate the occurrences of events. Thus assessing and establishing a good benefit risk ratio based on safety efficacy parameter of a particular drug becomes rather difficult. It also is the sponsor's responsibility to submit on a regular basis the PSURs, SUSARs of aspecific drug post approval for enabling the regulatory agencies to take a good judgement regarding the benefit risk profile of the drug both for an approved indication and off label use in pediatric population. As we have seen in this chapter that due to different stages of development in children, the drug therapy given at a particular stage might often elicit effects in a delayed manner and thus takes prolonged time for identification of the drug associated risks. Pharmaco-epidemiological studies thus become quint essential amongst the pediatric population.

Next we shall discuss the elderly or geriatric population. The country which has the maximum number of elderly population (60 and above 60 years of age) is US and Australia followed by Japan and France. The two main reasons for the reluctance of researchers to involve elderly people in clinical trials of drugs are that both multiple pathology and treatment with multiple drugs are common in the elderly population. The worry from the trial organisers' perspective is that interference from symptoms arising from concurrent disease or intercurrent illnesses may introduce bias and thus make the interpretation of adverse events more difficult. The elderly population at higher risks of developing either or couple of these diseases; *viz*: Cardiovascular, cerebrovascular, osteoarthrosis of joints and lower limbs, musculoskeletal disease. And thus treatment with multiple drugs may add to this interference, especially when there is concern about drug interactions and poor compliance. The list of drug therapy that the geriatric group is subjected to is endless. But some of them which are majorly prescribed are diuretics, followed by analgesics, hypnotics, sedatives, anxiolytics, drugs for rheumatism and gout, beta adrenoceptor antagonist. Considering this scenario, we believe that protocols should be specifically designed to account for comorbidity and treatment with multiple drugs. Compliance with protocols could be improved by involving pharmacists in counselling patients about the drug under investigation, and perhaps even visiting patients at home. Indeed the involvement of other support workers to coordinate the visits and investigations should be encouraged given the greater supervision necessary to ensure the accuracy of such trials in elderly people. It is important that we have sufficient information to be able to use drugs appropriately in elderly people, and that they should have the opportunity of benefiting from advances in medical knowledge and treatment. Approximately 50% of elderly populations take Over the counter (OTC) medication everyday. OTC medicines can interact with prescription medicines which may lead to adverse events. Besides, drug therapy in elderly is for long duration and includes polypharmacy. Underdose and overdose are equally the case whilst treatment of elderly population. Drug therapy is of longer duration that is more than 4–5 months because most of the disease conditions that elderly suffer are chronic. Especially the NSAID type of medications may thus cause serious problems because of regular intake which may lead to gastrointestinal bleeding. Secondly polypharmacy as stated also becomes essential to treat such chronic conditions, as there might be existing 2 or more diseases at the same time to the same patient and hence treating these conditions with a single drug becomes rather difficult.

Polypharmacy occurs due to one or all of the below mentioned reasons:

- Prevalence of many disease conditions that co-exist for a given patient.
- Single drug may not render the desired therapeutic response for the existing varied disease coditions.
- For ameliorating and giving relief from side effects. Many a times the intake of several drugs may lead to drug-drug interactions, which thus may cause an additional disease condition in a patient.
- Direct to consumer advertising by pharmaceutical companies may lead to polypharmacy in elderly lot.

Adverse reactions are caused due to intake of several drugs together *i.e.* polypharmacy. The magnitude and duration of action of one drug may be changed due to other drug. The reactions are precipitated sooner if there is a drug especially with higher toxicity rendering profile or low therapeutic index. This means the difference between the maximum safe concentration and minimum effective concentration is very less in such a drug which can lead to the crossing of blood levels above maximum safe concentration quite easily. Thus toxic effects can be experienced when such a drug react with other drug *i.e.* drug-drug interaction leading to precipitation of adverse reactions. Also these interactions are all the more possible if two or more drugs prscribed are incompatible with each other outright. This is more likely when these medications are prescribed by more than one physician. Further drug interactions may include drug interaction with another drug, with herbal supplements, with food, along with alcohol, milk etc. So also the food habits and lifestyle needs to be taken into consideration while prescribing medicines for the elderly.

Drug interactions may lead to alterations in the Absorption, Distribution, Metabolism and Excretion (ADME) of the drug. These are also known as Pharmaco-kinetic interactions. Thus when the ADME is either increased or decreased toxic effects are observed within the body. Each of the individual parameters are discussed in the context of geriatric population:

1. ***Absorption changes:***
   a. Solubility of a drug is decreased because of the presence of another drug and therefore the absorption is also reduced. This

leads to decrease in the systemic blood concentration of the drug thereby eliciting low or no therapeutic reponse.

b. *Absorption enhanced due to increased gastric motility:* When the gastric motility increases, proportionally absorption is also enhanced. *e.g.:* metoclopramide

c. *Absorption decreased due to decreased gastric motility:* When gastric motility decreases, there is an increase in absorption that is observed. *e.g.:* anticholinergics

d. *First pass metabolism of some drugs inhibited because of competition:* Presence of some drugs inhibit the first pass metabolism of a particular drug due to which the concentration in the blood is increased beyond the required level and thus elicits toxic effects.

Non selective Monoamine oxidase inhibitors (MAOIs) *e.g:* phenelzine competes for metabolism with tyramine that is found in cheese, tomatoes, chocolate and pseudoephedrine, direct and indirect sympathomimetic agents (Depicted as Fig. 1).

MAOI

↓ Reduce the metabolism of direct-indirect sympathomimetic agent

Direct or indirect sympathomimetic agent

↓

Large chunk of these amines reach the sympathetic nervous system

↓

Stimulate interneuronal release of Nor-adrenaline (NA)

↓

MAOI prevents break down of NA

↓

Results in headache, hypertension, excitement and delirium

Fig. 1: Depicting the effect of MAOI

Geriatric population: In case of the elderly, the rate and extent of absorption varies and becomes unpredictable. Changes such as reduction in acid secretion in the stomach, decreased gastric emptying and decreased gastrointestinal motility occur in such population. Albeit the changes that happen at the GIT end, an AUC Vs time profile, showed no major changes in a study conducted using oral and IV formulation for the elderly group.

2. ***Distribution changes:*** The Distribution changes take place when there are 2 or more drugs which compete for protein binding. If the two drugs are such that they are highyly protein bound, then they compete for binding to protein, such that free fraction or unbound amount of one of the drugs in the process increases and subsequently there is an increase in the concentration of the drug.

   For example:
   - Displacement of warfarin by NSAID, leads to greater anticoagulant effect of warfarin.
   - Displacement of tolbutamide from albumin by NSAID azapropazone.

   Geriatric population: Bioavailability of lipophilic drugs may increase in this population, because of lesser extraction of such drugs by liver due to age. Lipid soluble drugs are most widely distributed due to the increase in adipose tissues in elderly. On the contrary lipid insoluble drugs are present in higher concentrations in blood and have shorter elimination half lives also. Dose calculation should be carefully down while administering acidic drug to this sect of population. Especially acidic drugs which have low therapeutic index should be administered only after safe dose determination. This is because of the increased blood levels of such drugs due to a decrease in serum abumin levels which bind the acidic drugs to them. Likewise basic drugs' dose must be accurately determined because of their binding to the α-1-acid glycoprotein, that increases with age. In this case the dose of the drug that is actually given to a young adult if given to the elderly patient may lead to low or no therapeutic effect and increased elimination half life of the drug.

3. ***Metabolism changes:*** The triggering factor for drug metabolism changes, that could be either increased metabolism or decreased metabolism, is due to either inhibition or induction of the liver enzymes. In case of enzyme induction process, the time taken to for such changes to actually commence may be delayed to the extent of a week and hence identification of such reactions are difficult or rather linking the adverse reaction to the enzyme induction process because of the presence of other drug may not be done. Hence, this

point may be of great significance while peforming pharmacovigilance studies, so that no important signals per se are missed out during the process.

Few important cases are listed below which shows altered metabolism:

- Decreased efficacy of warfarin observed when administered along with barbiturates, due to induction of liver enzymes.
- Theophyllines clearance reduced by 39% when taken along with cimetidine due to inhibition of CYP isoenzyme
- Toxic plasma concentrations of procainamide observed due to consumption of the drug cimetidine concomitantly. This was due to the inhibition of isoenzyme CYP.
- Carbamazepine therapy leading to decreased efficacy of dihydropyridine calcium channel blocker.

Cytochrome P 450 (CYP) family is one of the major enzymes responsible for causing metabolism in humans. The CYP family is divided into 6 subfamilies:

a. CYP1A
b. CYP2A
c. CYP2C
d. CYP2D
e. CYP2E
f. CYP3A

Inhibition of CYP enzyme leads to a decreased metabolism of one of the given drugs. Food, diet and herbal supplements may also play a role in altered metabolism of drugs. Thus in case of polypharmacy which is very common amongst the geriatric population, can lead to several adverse reactions due to the inhibition of CYP isoenzymes which has the capability to metabolise several drugs. The drugs that inhibit CYP isoenzymes are: Cimetidine, fluconazole, erythromycin, clarithromycin, sulphonamides, ciprofloxacin, paroxetine, omeprazole and fluconazole. Cimetidine can cause reduced metabolism of β-adrenoceptor blockers, benzodiazepines, procainamide, theophylline, tricyclic antidepressants, phenytoin, oral anticoagulants and thereby lead to toxic concentrations of these drugs triggering the onset of adverse reactions. Care should be exercised especially when the drug is administered along with a drug which has the tendency to inhibit CYP leading to toxic concentrations of the unmetabolised drug. Thus drugs with low therapeutic index should not be consumed along with drugs which have inhibitory effect on CYP isoenzyme.

Geriatric population: One should be careful while giving a drug which might get metabolized to an active metabolite to an elderly patient. Because such metabolites may not be safe in the first pace and secondly such metabolite may also stay in the body for a very longer duration. It is generally observed with the elderly lot that the phase I oxidative metabolism, which renders an active drug less lipophilic, may be reduced. A lower hepatic clearance is observed in the patients with a lower hepatic blood flow.

4. ***Elimination changes:*** Excretion related changes related to a drug occur because of alterations in the excretion process. The various processes are penned down below:

   a. Glomerular filtration

   b. Tubular secretion

   c. Tubular reabsorption

   An increase in the drug excretion *via* glomerular filtration occurs due to displacement of bound drug. Competitive inhibition of tubular secretion as observed in the case of probencid *vs* penicillin leads to an increased drug concentration in the body and decreased drug excretion. Competition at the tubular site reabsorption leads to increased excretion of the drug from the body.

   We thus need to educate our elderly patients, our medical colleagues, and the public about the importance of including elderly patients in clinical research. However, more specifically, we suggest that paying more attention to the design of clinical trials of drugs could improve the reliability of the information yielded and provide a more practical approach to studying drug treatment in elderly people. Inevitably more financial resources will be necessary to achieve this goal.

   Geriatric population: Usual doses given to a young adult when given to an elderly may lead to toxic levels in the body. Creatinine clearance plays an important role in drug elimination and hence helps in determining the dose that needs to be given to an elderly thereby preventing toxic concentratons of the drug. A creatinine clearance of less than 40 ml per minute resulted in elevated plasma levels. ACE inhibitors, diuretics, NSAIDs and amino glycosides affect kidney functioning. It is also found that there is generally a decrement of 8 ml per minute of the glomerular filtration rate in every 10 years.

Since creatinine clearance plays a major role in deciding the dose that needs to be given to the elderly. The formula, popularly known as the Cockcroft formula, for calculating creatinine clearance is given as follows:

For male:

$$\text{Creatinine clearance} = \frac{1.23 \times (140 - \text{age}) \times \text{body weight(kg)}}{\text{Plasma creatinine } (\mu\text{moll}^{-1})}$$

For female:

$$\text{Creatinine clearance} = \frac{1.04 \times (140 - \text{age}) \times \text{body weight(kg)}}{\text{Plasma creatinine } (\mu\text{moll}^{-1})}$$

Further considering the Pharmacodynamic aspect of the drug behaviour, adverse reactions are also caused due to the altered pharmacodynamic aspect of a particular drug when administered concurrently with another drug. Pharmacodynamics is the study of the action of the drug on the body. Such adverse reactions are the result of a drug-drug interaction. Adverse reactions occur generally when there is an enhanced effect due to interaction of two different drugs.

Below mentioned is a list of adverse reactions due to variations in the pharmacodynamic aspect of a drug because of the interaction with another drug:

- Butyrophenones and phenothiazines interact with anticholinergic drugs leading to urinary hesitancy, dry mouth, confusion, constipation.
- Digoxin may interact with loop diuretics or thiazides and cause arrhythmias. This is because of diuretics induced hypokalaemia.
- Quinolones may interact with NSAIDs that may lead to seizures.
- Potassium sparing diuretics may interact with potassium supplements and ACE inhibitors leading to renal dysfunction and hyperkalaemia. ACE inhibitors with NSAIDs also showed similar effects.

- It was found both in case of phenytoin, cyclosporine, tricyclic antidepressants carbamazepine and theophylline that an interaction with enzyme inhibitors may lead to an enhanced effect of the original drugs and a reduced clearance.

Drugs like calcium antagonists, antidepressants, ciclosporin, theophylline, thyroxine and corticosteroids show reduced effects on interaction with enzyme inducers. They show reduced effects because of their increased clearance.

Finding suitable elderly people to participate in clinical trials is a challenge. Resource limitations, cost factors, or the race to establish efficacy for a new drug are common reasons to use a cleaner population in the early stages of a trial. However, to get the most value, researchers argue, a drug or therapy needs to be tested by the people who will use it. Electronic Prescribing will help as the connecting link between prescription and clinical outcomes will be identifiable.

It is recommended that researchers make every attempt to include older patients with co-morbidities in studies of therapies that are likely to be used in this segment of the population. In addition, they recommend that the FDA, funding agencies and policy makers institute guidelines to encourage the inclusion of older adults in such studies. In today's scenario, wherein the geriatric population is increasing also simultaneously the nation's health care expenditures are elevating. And only more will join the group 10 years down the line. This creates a pressing need for more geriatric research and clinical guidelines for physicians who treat this growing population.

The next population that is of special significance in pharmacovigilance studies is the pregnant women population. Interestingly, the medication consumed in such population and the adverse reaction that followed marked a new turning point in the world of clinical trials and pharmacovigilance. Thalidomide disaster was one of the major historic events which involved consumption of thalidomide, a sedative by pregnant women which eventually showed its adverse repercussions as severe congenital anomalies in many of the offspring. Albeit it was safe for the mother it proved fatal to the foetus. Pharmacovigilance studies in this population thus become quintessential. Another reason that's makes PV studies so significant in pregnant women is the number of medications or drug therapy they are exposed in the course of gestation. The number of medications that this population is expsosed to, is all the more than observed before conception. Spontaneous abortions, long term post natal functional deficits or learning disabilities with the off spring are all reasons which need attention for this population to be thoroughly studied whilst they are exposed to therapies. However programs STEPS and SMART have been designed exclusively for the prevention of pregnancy exposure to teratogens and to market such high risk teratogens in a sensible way. STEP is program to prevent the pregnancy exposure to thalidomide by following stringent drug dispensing through registered clinicians, pharmacists. Further also the women of child bearing age are thoroughly monitored and educated about this program. Likewise SMART is an initiative taken for the teratogen isotretinoin which is a pregnancy prevention program. Further for isotretinoin, a program called iPLEDGE is conducted which is to prevent exposure of this teratogen to pregnant women. Below mentioned is a list of resources from where the reports pertaining to drug safety during pregnancy can be obtained.

Table 1: Resources: Drug Safety Reports During Pregnancy

S.no	*Resources*	*Information*	*Limitations*
1.	Clinician case reports	Published in medical literature.	• Investigator or publication bias due to spontaneous reporting • Exposure of number of pregnancies unknown. • Number of infants affected with malformations due to drug exposure from these pregnancies is unknown.
2.	Centralized adverse event reporting systems (AERSs)	• Manufacturers and distributors of FDA approved pharmaceuticals need to report events to the FDA.	• Under Medwatch program, HCPs need to report adverse events to FDA. • Consumers directly to FDA or manufacturers • Have not been helpful in identifying new teratogens. • Investigator or publication bias in reporting the number and types of actual events due to spontaneous reporting.

Table 1: *(Contd...)*

Table 1: *(Contd...)*

S.no	*Resources*	*Information*	*Limitations*
			• Lack of motivation in reporting the events caused by a particular product if it has been in market for a long time. • Exposure of number of pregnancies unknown. • Number of infants affected or not affected with malformations due to drug exposure from these pregnancies is unknown. • Reporting those events which have outcomes that are rare and extremely severe and less likely to report events that are common and milder.
3.	Pregnancy drug exposure registries	• Spontaneous reporting of exposed pregnancies by the HCP who initiates contact with the registry. • In some registries the outcome and exposure data is collected from the pregnant woman.	• Selection bias possible because of spontaneous reporting. • Difficulty in identifying an appropriate comparison group and thus outcomes in exposed pregnancies are many times compared with externally derived reference rates for general population. • Because of various HCPs and consumers reporting pregnancy outcomes, there is quite a chance of outcomes being mis-classified like major congenital anomalies with regards to accurate and complete diagnosis and/or suspected etiology. On the other hand subtle teratogenic effects may go amiss, because the HCP did not identify it and thus is not reported to the registry.
4.	Birth defects monitoring or surveillance systems	Population/hospital based surveillance systems for identifying anomalies for measuring their patterns and then accordingly responding	-------

Table 1: *(Contd...)*

Table 1: *(Contd...)*

S.no	*Resources*	*Information*	*Limitations*
		to this unusual pattern of events.	
5.	Birth defects case control studies	• Classical hypothesis testing case control designs. • Ongoing case control surveillance.	• Being a retrospective study generally, there might be chances of missing out on medications exposure by mothers while recalling. • Possible bias in the information regarding therapy exposed to by mothers of malformed infants and mothers of nonmalformed infants. • A potential congenital anomaly which is unusual in nature may not be recorded because it may not fall in the database of expected anomalies in this particular study.
6.	Large cohort studies	Open cohorts that are ongoing population based, hospital or health insurer based.	• Collaborative prenatal project with lesser populaiton exposed unable to detect weak to moderate associations of risk factors with congenital malformations but the swedish registry with a larger pool of patient population exposed conducted for 25 years was able to detect those associations.
7.	Small cohort studies	Conducted by teratology information services, North America and Europe.	• Sample size less ranging between 100 and 200. • Selection bias with regards to recruitment of subject, since this based on spontaneous callers.
8.	Database linkage studies	Medicaid database links maternal prescription records to pediatric billing records.	• No subject contact, thus cannot be ensured that the prescription to the mother was consumed by her. • Misclassification of outcomes depending on the quality of records.

One advantage of centralized adverse event reporting systems (AERSs) is that reports of adverse events can be obtained from various resources abiding by timelines. Although as mentioned above, this method has been inadept in identifying new teratogens, but it has proved beneficial in probing more into the case once a teratogen of a new kind has been identified by other methods. Also some of the neonatal complications presented by late pregnancy exposure to anti-depressants identified by the case reports and case studies were confirmed by the AERS data.

Further in prospective type of registries approach can provide inputs on temporal association between the drug exposure and the outcome. Also comparison of the congenital anomaly rates to the reference group can be done in registries because of the defined or fixed denominator of women exposed to such registries.

Birth defects case control studies follow two approaches; *viz:* classical hypothesis testing case control designs and ongoing case control surveillance for drug induced congenital anomalies. Considering the classical hypothesis testing case control designs, the possible link between the risk factor and the observed birth defect in the form of a congenital anomaly is observed between the 2 groups, *i.e.* the cases and control group. And accordingly the probability factor is calculated. Like for example: the occurrence of facial nerve paralysis and the use of misoprostol in the first trimester of pregnancy. However in the second approach as the name suggests, an ongoing case control surveillance includes a study which is made ongoing so as to collect a large repository of data. Here there is no fixed drug or outcome about which the study is done. This focuses on the gathering exposure data and the malformed and non malformed information on infants from cases and control groups. This study is directed towards confirming the malformed cases and also non malformed infants are taken as controls for the study. Here the genetic susceptibility is tested in some instances for which DNA sampling is also done. Moderate or lower concentration teratogens causing malformations are identified in this case. This study also has the potential of identifying risks associated with newly marketed medication because of the ongoing nature of the study.

Thus bagged with several advantages, the methods of Pharmacovigilance in detecting drug safety or the link between the risk factor and the observed congenital anomaly/malformation has its own set of limitations though. As it is observed above, the major limitation is the less sample size to which the drug is exposed. Besides, the setback regarding methods incapable of identifying teratogenic effects related to a new drug molecule. Again several other concerns such as irregualr use of a particular medication, the birth defect not being unique, or difficulty in recognizing such defects are drawbacks still being observed. Also prospective studies as seen in registries are a limitation that needs though to be overruled. Because the mother may not be able to recall the medications or dose used during the gestation period in a prospective study. Therefore, there needs to be a systematic approach to streamline and channelise various methods of pharmacovigilance in an appropriate manner or a proper collaborative approach between the available methods need to be done so as to overcome the above mentioned limitations. If this is taken care and done in a co-ordinated and timely manner, it can be a boon to delivering healthy offsprings.

In the Pregnant population, to involve such patients in the trial is a risk, both to the mother and the foetus. Also getting the exact scenario of the adverse reactions pertaining to a drug is difficult in such a circumstance due to the random Absorption, Distribution, Metabolism and Excretion (ADME) patterns. But this problem can be trouble shooted by considering pharmacokinetic studies done alongside appropriate calculations of the dose on healthy volunteers. This will help also to arrive at a safe medication with an appropriate dose which falls well within the therapeutic window.

Thus this chapter emphasises on how significant it is to have a preliminary testing of the new drug moiety at initial stages *i.e* prior to marketing during clinical trials. This can thus help in deciding the appropriate dose, the regular hazards that are possible to occur and also the interaction of the drug molecule with other frequently consumed medication in such population.

9

PSURs and SUSARs

The periodic safety update report for marketed drugs (PSUR) is a stand-alone document that allows a periodic but comprehensive assessment of the worldwide safety data of a marketed drug or biological product. Council for International Organizations of Medical Sciences (CIOMS) II working group was instrumental in developing the concept of PSUR. This was done so as to reduce the burden of manufacturers regarding submission of different kinds of reports to various local regulatory bodies in various formats. Thus to avoid the cumbersome process of submitting reports in different formats, criteria and timelines, the initiative was taken. The PSUR being a worldwide safety information of a medicinal product post authorization, can be an important source for the identification of new safety signals, a means of determining changes in the benefit-risk profile, an effective means of risk communication to regulatory authorities and an indicator for the need for risk management initiatives, as well as a tracking mechanism monitoring the effectiveness of such initiatives. For these reasons, the PSUR can be an important pharmacovigilance tool. Critical evaluation of the risk-benefit balance of the product in light of the new information is presented by the marketing authorization holders. This evaluation decides if there needs to be further evaluation done and also if there needs to be changes done with regards marketing authorization and/or product information. PSUR gives information on the overall safety profile of the drug. The regulatory authorities can thus figure out from a PSUR, if the product's safety has undergone modifications from the time of its authorisation or is it the same. And in case there are any drastic changes which relate to the so called adverse reation, signal, then there can be call taken by the regulatory authority whether any changes are to be done regarding the product information usage.

The concept developed from the Council for International Organizations of Medical Sciences (CIOMS) Working Group II report (CIOMS, 1992). The publication of that report was initiated in 1989, when quite a few countries had requirements for periodic safety updates. Both foreign and domestic data had to be presented according to different inclusion criteria, formats and time intervals in accordance with the request made by the individual local regulatory authorities. However, the number of reports that had to be produced was placing a tremendous administrative encumberance on manufacturers.

Numerous steps are involved in the PSUR process including: intake of adverse drug reaction information, case processing, data retrieval, data analysis, and medical review and risk assessment. These processes are heavily reliant on the availability of adequate resources. An overarching principle throughout the PSUR process is the need for a proactive approach in order to identify the critical steps in the process and to have a clear understanding of the consequences of any critical 'mis-step'. With this information comes appropriate planning, building quality into each step of the PSUR process and monitoring performance will maximise the likelihood of generating a quality report. A poor quality report that will give little insight into emerging safety signals or provide misleading information that can adversely affect public health is the resultant of any failure of a key PSUR process. A pragmatic approach that will avoid or minimize these pitfalls includes the following: adequate resource planning, training, development of 'scripts' designed to maximize the capture of key information for medically important reactions, standardized and harmonized Medical Dictionary for Regulatory Activities (MedDRA) coding procedures, pre-specified search criteria for data retrieval, ongoing medical review, and metrics to evaluate the effectiveness and efficiencies of these processes. With these quality measures in place, the utility of the PSUR as an effective pharmacovigilance tool is bettered.

CIOMS II not only took initiative in coming up with the theme of PSUR for a more balanced and harmonized approach of saftey report submission across countries but it also listed the contents for PSURs and the way in which the format should look like. Also the concept of an International Birth Date (IBD) was introduced for the first time. IBD signifies the date of first approval in the world. The PSUR has now been adopted in many European countries, Japan and the United States. It is emerging as a gold standard of safety evaluation for marketed drugs and an important pharmacovigilance tool. The PSUR also helps in optimizing the use of a product. This is done by assessing if the safety profile is the same from the time of its approval or has it changed after its authorization and to specify whether changes should be made to product information to optimise the use of a product. Thus an overall evaluation is done by PSUR in a periodic way. Because of the obvious limitations of clinical trials like unreal clinical situation, limited number of patient pool, and lesser duration of drug exposure, a periodic assessment post drug approval, *i.e.* when the drug arrives in the market is essential. Being an unreal clinical situation, clinical trials have inclusion and exclusion criteria. After a product is launched, it may be used by patients not studied in clinical trials, for example children, the elderly, pregnant or breastfeeding women or patients with comorbidities such as hepatic or renal disease. After approval, a drug becomes available for instant and direct use in large populations, so rare adverse drug reactions (ADRs) can be more effortlessly identified and delayed onset reactions is identified too, now because the drug is used for a prolonged duration in real life scenario and the drugs also become available for indefinite use (unless prescribing information indicates otherwise).

Mentioned below are the various scenarios, wherein the PSUR may be submitted in a different format. They are as mentioned below:

One Report for Products Containing One Active Substance Authorised to One Marketing Authorisation Holder

A given marketing authorisation holder (MAH), may submit a single PSUR for all the formulations (syrups, tablets, capsules etc), of various strengths (for example: 500 mg and 250 mg Ibuprofen) containing the same Active Pharmaceutical Ingredient (API). Also the formulations containing the same API for different indications may be submitted by the MAH in the same PSUR. Thus, all dosage forms of varying strength as well as indications for a given pharmacologically active substance for medicinal products authorised to one marketing authorisation holder (MAH) may be covered in one PSUR. Within the single PSUR, separate presentations of data for different dosage forms, indications or populations (*e.g.* children versus adults) may be suitable.

Products Authorised to More than One MAH

If there are more than one MAHs' for the same product, each MAH should submit their own PSUR. Even if there are more than one MAH for a given product in the same country, then individual PSURs need to be submitted by each manufacturer. In case of a licenser-licensee kind of arrangements where the product manufacturing is contract research manufacturing, the safety issues concerned with the products must be clearly and transparently discussed and the same needs to be sorted out during PSUR submission. This will help in efficient safety reporting in such cases and no relevant information is in the process missed out.

Combination Products

This section discusses the PSUR submissions for combination products *i.e.* two different APIs', which have separate authorizations. In this scenario, either a separate PSUR should be submitted for the combination formulation or the combinations' detail or safety report can be included as a separate presentation for in same PSUR, which is that of one of the active components of the combination. However, it has to be borne in mind that the cross referencing of all essential PSURs is a must.

General Scope of Information

The relevant clinical and non-clinical safety data that is included as a part of PSUR should be those set of data/information which should cover only the period of the report (interval data). The exception to this rule includes, data regarding regulatory status information on authorisation applications plus renewals if any and data on serious, unlisted ADRs, which should be provided for both the period in question and as cumulative summary tabulations starting from the IBD. A listed ADR is one whose nature, severity, specificity and outcome are consistent with the company core safety information (CCSI). And unlisted ADR is one whose nature, severity, specificity and outcome are inconsistent with the company core safety information (CCSI). A serious ADR is defined as any untoward medical occurrence that at any dose results in death, is life threatening, requires in-patient hospitalisation or prolongation of existing hospitalisation, results in persistent or significant disability/incapacity or is a congenital abnormality/birth defect. The PSUR consists of safety information that is obtained from various sources. These include spontaneous reports of adverse events from different countries, the literature, clinical trials, registries, regulatory ADR databases and important animal findings (preclinical data). All adverse spontaneous experiences should be assumed to be ADRs; unless diagnosed other wise by a Health Care Profesisonal (HCP). In case of clinical trial and literature cases, only those reported not related to the drug by both the reporter and the manufacturer/sponsor should be excluded. A paramount risk is associated with lack of efficacy cases observed in cases where the drug is used in treatment of life-threatening conditions and for certain other medicinal products, such as contraceptives and vaccines. This type of cases may thus pose a serious safety issue to the patient. Such cases should therefore be discussed in the PSUR.

Preparation of PSURS According to the IBD

IBD is the date on which first marketing authorisation is granted for a product granted to any company in any country in the world. For administrative convenience, if desired by the MAH, the IBD can be designated as the last day of the same month. When the CIOMS II proposals (CIOMS became operative since 1949) were first incorporated into European regulations, they were modified to include the concept of a European birth date rather than an IBD. This meant that PSURs currently scheduled to the IBD had to be rescheduled to the first European approval date – which seemed to be defying the drive for harmonisation. However it was good news, when ICH E2C (which came into existence later than CIOMS *i.e.* in 1990s) reverted to the IBD for scheduling reports, so now the European birth date is the same as the

IBD for medicinal products first authorised in the European Union (EU), and the MAH may use the IBD to determine data-lock points (DLPs) in Europe. The DLP is the date designated as the cut-off for data to be included in a PSUR.

Frequency of Reporting

Every PSUR should include the period since the last update report and should be submitted within 60 days of the last DLP. The local regulatory requirements decide on the need for a report and the frequency of report submission to authorities. The age of a medicinal product and related safety issues with regards the product on the market may influence this process. Receiving authorisations for a relatively new product launched in the market at different times in different countries is a norm in the initial years of product launch. It is during this early period that harmonisation of reporting is particularly important. Once a product has been marketed for several years, the need for a comprehensive PSUR and the frequency of reporting may be reviewed, depending on local regulations or requests while maintaining one IBD for all regulatory authorities. In Europe, for example, the last 6-month PSUR should be provided at the first renewal while for subsequent renewals either a single 5-year PSUR or separate 6 month or yearly PSURs covering 5 years, together with a PSUR bridging summary report, are required.

Restarting the Clock

Apart from initial approval for the active substance, further approvals may be granted by the regulatory bodies for reasons including new indications, dosage forms, routes of administration or populations other than for populations for which the active substance was initially authorised. Other population here means, it may have been contraindicated for pregnant women, wherein the consequent approvals may be done for use in pregnant women as per the requirement. This generally happens in situation wherein on a later date, from the relevant safety trials, reports and analysis, the drug is found useful also in the pregnant population. The probable consequences for the safety profile of new types and extent of population exposure should be discussed between the regulatory authorities and the MAH because they may influence the requirements for periodic reporting. While submitting an amendment of the PSUR submission cycle to the regulatory authority, the applicant should submit a logical reason as part of the application for a marketing authorisation.

Reference Safety Information

The listing of all the relevant safety information wih regards a drug marketed in varios countries worldwide is done in the CCSI which is derived from the company core data sheet (CCDS). The CCSI forms the basis for determining whether an ADR is listed or unlisted, as opposed to labelled or unlabelled. If the ADR reported is found in the approved product information for a given country, the event is considered labelled. If not, it is unlabelled. The European Summary of Product Characteristics (SPC) or locally approved product information continues to be the reference document upon which labelledness (or expectedness) is based for the purpose of local expedited post-authorisation safety reporting, so labelledness is country-specific. On the contrary, Listedness is uniform across all countries, and it is listedness that must be determined for the PSUR.

Description of the Reaction

The reaction terms mentioned in the PSUR is often derived from the standard terminology used by the reporting MAH. Medical Dictionary for Regulatory Activities (MedDRA) is used in many cases. MedDRA was developed in the early 1990s under the auspices of the ICH and is an important step towards the standardisation of terminology regarding the registering, documenting and safety monitoring of medical products. MedDRA has been discussed in detail before. MedDRAs use in spontaneous reporting systems is currently a regulatory requirement in some countries, and it is widely used in the preparation of PSURs. In November 1997, the FDA replaced its spontaneous reporting system and its conventional dictionary, the Coding Symbols for a Thesaurus of Adverse Reaction Terms, with the new adverse events reporting system and the MedDRA terminology. MedDRA is also a key part of the electronic database systems used by European and Japanese authorities.

Regulatory Requirements

ICH E2C covers the topic clinical safety data management and periodic safety update reports. ICH E2C along with its addendum has been adopted by the Japanese Ministry of Health, Labour and Welfare. The US Food and Drug Administration (FDA) has also introduced periodic reporting requirements based on ICH E2C, and published a guidance for industry in February 2004 (FDA, 2004). ICH E2C has thus made its mark in all three ICH regions. Nevertheless, the reporting requirements in those regions differ:

- In the EU, Council Directive 93/39/EEC and Council Regulation 2309/93 require that reports be submitted every 6 months for the first 2 years '[after authorisation]' annually for the three following years and then five yearly after the first renewal;
- In the United States, the FDA requires quarterly reports during the first 3 years, then annual reports, and
- In Japan, the authorities require a survey on a cohort of a few thousand patients established by a certain number of identified institutions during the 6 years following authorisation. Systematic information on this cohort, taking into account a precise denominator, must be reported annually. Regarding other marketing experience, adverse reactions which are non-serious, but both mild in severity and unlabelled, must be reported every 6 months for 3 years and annually thereafter.

Significance of a PSUR

A stand alone global standardized document that can be used world-wide for:

- Identification of new safety signals
- Identification of changes to benefit-risk profile of medical product:
  a. Change in product label
  b. Change in product name, product package or promotional material
  c. Need for risk management initiatives
  d. Withdrawal of the product from market
- Monitoring effectiveness of risk management initiatives.

Information in PSUR

Irrespective of the marketing status, PSURS needs to be submitted for all registered products. Multiple reports are not essential in cases where there are different products containing the same Active Pharmaceutical Ingredient (API). Single report will suffice but it needs to be licensed by one MA holder. All relevant information including all formulations, dosage forms and indications of a particular API needs to be incorporated in the PSUR. Albeit separate presentations for different dosage forms, indications and populations needs to be presented but the PSUR must also contain a summary which presents a combined data.

Instances where there is a product containing two different API's which are registered separately, PSURs may be submitted as one single report for a fixed combination or separate reports for each substance. But care needs to be taken to cross reference all the relevant PSURs. Every pertinent clinical and non clinical safety data should include only the period of the report with the exception of the authorization status information for initial and renewal applications and data on serious unlisted adverse reactions. For clinical study and literature cases, all adverse events reported spontaneously should be considered adverse reactions. The spontaneous reports where the adverse events are declared as unrelated to the product by the reporter and MA holder are not considered into the adverse reactions category.

The data from the following sources needs to be included in the PSUR by the MA holder:

1. ***Direct reports to MA holder***
   a. Spontaneous notifications from healthcare professionals
   b. MA holder sponsored clinical studies or compassionate use studies
   c. Spontaneous reports from consumers/patients
2. Literature reports
3. ADR reporting systems of regulatory authorities
   a. Spontaneous notifications
   b. Nonspontaneous notifications
4. Other sources of data
   a. Reports of adverse reactions exchanged between licensor-licensee

b. Data in special registries

c. Reports created by poison control centers

d. Epidemiological database

Intervals of PSUR Reporting Requirements

For all the medicinal products, PSUR needs to be submitted at following intervals. The PSUR submission starts from the time of authorisation. Following are the time lines for submission of a PSUR:

- Immediately upon request
- Atleast 6 monthly after authorisation and until placing on the market.
- Atleast 6 monthly for first two years after being placed on the market.
- Annually for the subsequent two years
- Thereafter at three yearly intervals.

A PSUR summary bridging report (BSR) serves the purpose whenever MAH decides to submit multilple six monthly reports. The cut of date for the data to be included in a PSUR is Data lock point (DLP). DLP is set according to the European birth date (EBD) or International birth date (IBD). DLP is the cut off date for the data to be included in the report. IBD is the date on which the first approval of product happened in the world. It is necessary that the MAH submits the report not later than 2 months from the DLP. Every period needs to cover the period of time since the last update report.

DLP for generic products is not the same as that for innovators. For generic products the process of PSUR submission is simpler. The submission intervals are eased out unless there are any potential safety issues with the medicinal product during the safety assessment. The submissions can be done directly from the three yearly time cycle in line with the innovator product. This is in accordance with the European agreement. But there needs to be a request made in the registration dossier which will be agreed as a part of MA approval. If this is not done then there will the usual 6 monthly interval for two years, annually for two years and then three yearly PSUR reports after that, applicable even in case of generic products.

Table of Contents of PSUR

1. Introduction
2. World wide market authorization
3. Update of regulatory authority or MAH actions taken for safety issues.
4. Changes in reference safety information
5. Patient exposure
6. Presentation of individual case histories
7. Studies
8. Other information
9. Overall safety evaluation
10. Conclusion
11. ***Appendix:*** Company core data sheet and consumer reports
12. ***Appendix II:*** Marketing authorisation status
13. Line listing of case reports
14. Summary tabulation of events

Title: Title page should contain a statement on the confidentiality of the data and conclusions in the report.

Executive summary: This page should contain a brief outline providing the description of the most important information.

Introduction: This part includes a brief summary of drug's characteristics. It describes the products/formulations that are incorporated and excluded, outlines the pharmacology of the product, its indications (both marketed and in clinical trials) and any co-licensing agreements. The data about the drug from the last PSUR report to the data lock point. The number represented by the report, for example 1st periodic safety update report, 6th PSUR report etc.

World wide marketing authorization: This includes a table representative of the countries where the drug was approved and the countries where there was lack of approval etc. This should include a short précis of the worldwide marketing authorisation status and a crossreferencing to an appendix in which the cumulative approvals (and renewal dates) are tabulated in chronological sequence is done. This table should also include lack of approval, relevant explanations from regulatory authorities and withdrawals by the company for efficacy or safety reasons.

Update of regulatory authority or MAH actions taken for safety reasons: This section includes detail which is mentioned below:

- Marketing authorization, withdrawal or suspension
- Failure to obtain marketing re-authorization or authorization renewal
- Restrictions on distribution
- Dosage modification/formulation changes
- Withdrawal from market
- Suspension of clinical trials etc.
- Changes in target population or indications

The update should highlight and detail regarding the safety-related reasons that led to the actions described and appends the appropriate documentation including any communication with healthcare professionals.

Changes in reference safety information: This segment summarizes the changes essential to be made in the company core safety information (CCSI) from that existing in the current CCSI.

The changes in reference safety information section refers to changes in the CCSI. The CCDS, which incorporates the CCSI, should be included as an appendix. If no CCDS is available, a national SPC can be used. A covering letter should discuss meaningful differences between the CCSI and local datasheets and comment on the consequences for safety evaluations and for actions proposed or initiated.

Patient exposure: This deals with the disclosure of the quantity of medication exposed to the patients. It includes, for example:

- Number of bottles of medications distributed
- Number of tablets sold
- Number of prescriptions written

Presentation of individual case histories: This section incorporates listings, tabulation of AEs and analysis of all case histories.

1. This section incorporates listings of all the AE's reported by a patient of the most serious listed first. These are as mentioned below:
   - All serious reactions, non serious unlisted reactions from spontaneous notifications.
   - All serious reactions (attributable to drug either by sponsor or investigator) available from studies or named patient (compassionate) use.
   - All serious reactions, non serious unlisted reactions from literature
   - All serious reactions from regulatory authorities
2. Tabulation of AE's including tabulation of all non serious listed reactions.
3. Analysis of individual case histories. This is done to carefully detect the AE's and their occurrence rationale with the medicinal product.

Studies: Here the studies done on patients with the medicinal product are taken into consideration. But completed studies are considered to observe if there is any new safety related information.

Other information: This includes any information pertaining to the new efficacy of the medicinal product and breaking late news etc.

Overall safety evaluation: A succinct analysis is done taking into account all the accumulated data from various sources *viz:* spontaneous notifications, clinical studies, literature, compassionate use etc. Also any late breaking news followed by MAH's evaluation of the significance indicating a change in the benefit-risk profile of the drug is taken into account for the analysis. Additionally there are some more essential parameters which will add on to making a complete analysis. The parameters are as mentioned below:

- Certain specific populations are considered such as: the elderly, pediatric and pregnant women.
- Drug interactions
- Overdose

- Long term effects of a particular drug.
- Lack of efficacy pertaining to a drug.

Conclusion: The safety findings that are different than that included in the current reference safety information must be indicated in this part. This section should also be indicative of what actions were taken or will be taken in the future in terms of risk management initiatives. Also the amendments with regard to the Company Core Safety Information (CCSI) needs to be indicated.

Appendix: This section must contain Company Core Data Sheet (CCDS) and consumer reports.

The periodic safety update report for marketed drugs (PSUR) is an essential pharmacovigilance tool, which is a periodic but comprehensive assessment of the worldwide safety data of a marketed drug or biological product. Thus new safety signals, a means of determining changes in the benefit-risk profile, an effective means of risk communication to regulatory authorities and an indicator for the need for risk management initiatives can be gathered from a PSUR. Adverse drug reaction information collection, data retrieval, case processing, data analysis, medical review and risk assessment are the important aspects of PSUR processing. Identifying the critical steps in the process and to have a clear understanding of the consequences of any critical 'mis-step' are vital steps in PSUR process. This is because misleading information can adversely affect public health. Standardised and harmonised Medical Dictionary for Regulatory Activities (MedDRA) coding procedures, pre-specified search criteria for data retrieval, ongoing medical review, and metrics to evaluate the effectiveness and efficiencies of these processes are significant elements during PSUR compiling and processing.

SUSARS: Is defined as a Suspected Unexpected Serious Adverse Reaction.

To comprehend SUSARS and its regulations with clarity, below mentioned is a list of definitions along with some comments:

Adverse event (AE): Any untoward medical occurrence in a patient or clinical trial subject administered a medicinal product and which does not necessarily have a causal relationship with this treatment. Thus, an adverse event can therefore be any unfavourable and unintended sign (including an abnormal laboratory finding), symptom, or disease temporarily associated with the use of an investigational medicinal product, whether or not considered related to the investigational medicinal product.

Adverse reaction: Any untoward and unintended responses to an investigational medicinal product related to any dose administered. All adverse events judged by either the reporting investigator or the sponsor as having a reasonable causal relationship to a medicinal product qualify as adverse reactions. The expression "reasonable causal relationship" means to convey in general that there is evidence or argument to suggest a causal relationship.

Unexpected adverse reaction: An adverse reaction, the nature or severity of which is not consistent with the applicable product information (*e.g.* investigator's brochure for an unauthorised investigational product or summary of product characteristics for an authorised product). When the outcome of the adverse reaction is not consistent with the applicable product information this adverse reaction should be considered as unexpected.

Serious adverse event (SAE) or serious adverse reaction (SAR) or suspected unexpected serious adverse reaction (SUSAR)

Any AE, AR or UAR that at any dose:

- results in death
- is life-threatening
- requires hospitalisation or prolongation of existing hospitalisation
- results in persistent or significant disability or incapacity
- consists of a congenital anomaly or birth defect

Thus in deciding seriousness, medical judgement needs to be exercised in inferring whether an adverse event/reactions is serious in other situations. Important adverse events/reactions that are not immediately life-threatening or do not result in death or hospitalisation but may jeopardise the subject or may require intervention to prevent one of the other outcomes listed in the definition above, should also be considered serious. Life-threatening in the definition of a serious adverse event or serious adverse reaction refers to an event in which the subject was at risk of death at the time of event. It does not refer to an event which hypothetically might have caused death if it were more severe. The definition of seriousness above reflect the definition used in the EU Directive, and from EudraCT guidance. 'Other important medical condition' is taken from ICH E2A.

Risk assessment: In case of clinical trials depending on the risk associated, it may be reasonable to collect one or more of the following:

- All AEs (serious and/or non-serious)
- Only SAEs
- All ARs (serious and/or non-serious)
- Only SARs
- Only SAEs and SARs All AEs/ARs of a certain grade of severity, graded using standard toxicity grading scales such as CTCAE, WHO or Division of AIDS.
- Safety critical or 'notable' events

The proposed safety recording, notification and reporting procedures should be detailed in the trial protocol and will be reviewed by the MHRA during the CTA assessment. Three very important parameters that need to be considered while evaluating an adverse event are:

- Assessment of Seriousness
- Assessment of Causality
- Assessment of Expectedness

These factors are further discussed in detail below. For the completeness of the evalution of the safety report all three parameters should be appropriately and meticulously assessed. Thus taking into consideration only the seriousness of the event in hand is not enough. It is equally important that the suspectedness or causality of the adverse event with regards the drug is established and also at the same time one more thing needs to be considered *i.e* if the adverse event was expected or not. Like for instance, in case of fatal incidences like death, the event is very serious, but again was it caused due to the medication or was it due to previous medical history of the patient, or was it due to concomitant medications needs to established also.

Assessment of seriousness: This is based on the regulatory definitions of seriousness. These definitions should be included in the trial protocol.

Any AE, AR or UAR that at any dose:

- results in death
- is life-threatening*
- requires hospitalisation or prolongation of existing hospitalisation
- results in persistent or significant disability or incapacity
- consists of a congenital anomaly or birth defect

The term "severe" is often used to describe the intensity (clinical severity) of a specific event. This is not the same as "serious," which is a regulatory definition based on patient/event outcome or action criteria. For example, a headache may be severe but not serious while a minor stroke may be serious but not severe.

Assessment of causality

- A clinical assessment of whether the adverse event is likely to be related to the trial drug.
- All adverse events judged as having a reasonable suspected causal relationship (*e.g.* definitely, probably or possibly related) to the study drug are considered to be adverse reactions.
- The local investigator responsible for the patient may be best placed to make the immediate assessment of causality, distinguishing suspected adverse reactions from unrelated adverse events.
- Where there are two assessments of an event, the sponsor cannot downgrade the causality assessment made by the investigator. In the case of a difference of opinion on causality, both assessments are recorded, and the 'worst case' assessment is used for reporting purposes.

Assessment of expectedness: The evaluation of expectedness is based on knowledge of the adverse reaction and any relevant product information. The list of expected events should be based on:

- The Summary Product Characteristics (SPC) for the products under investigation for a licensed drug or
- The investigator's brochure (IB) for a non-licensed drug.

Where a study is taking place in more than one country, using a licensed medicine with different SPCs around the globe, a single SPC and labelling information (the most comprehensive) should be selected as the reference document for all trial sites, and this should be documented in the protocol.

Assessment of adverse events

- The EC guidance document ENTR/CT3 suggests that the local investigator assesses seriousness and causality while the sponsor assesses expectedness. However, the Regulations allow the duties of sponsors to be delegated, including to investigators.
- Whatever decision is made for a given clinical trial it is vital that the arrangement is documented in the trial protocol and/or SOPs in any agreements or contracts between the sponsor and the investigator.
- The most appropriate person or group to evaluate expectedness will depend on how the clinical trial is organised.
- There is no legal requirement for two independent assessments of an event.

Assessment of adverse events in blinded trials: Maintenance of blinding can be crucial to the integrity of a trial. Hence, systems for SUSAR and SAR reporting should, as far as possible, maintain blinding of individual clinicians and of trials staff involved in the day-to-day running of the trial. In case of blinded trials involving a placebo and an active drug, the investigator should evaluate SAEs for causality and expectedness as though the patient was on an active drug. Only cases that are considered serious, unexpected and possibly, probably or definitely related (*i.e.* SUSARs) would have to be unblinded for reporting to the regulatory authority and ethics committee. In case of blinded trials involving two active drugs, the investigator making the assessment might be able to state that if the patient were on drug A the event would be causal and/or unexpected, but if on drug B it would be expected. If the event were unexpected for either of the active drugs, the case should be unblinded by the individual charged with unblinding, who would then classify the event accordingly. It may be that individuals who are not directly involved in the management of the trial could perform unblinding (for example, in a trials unit, staff working on a separate trial might undertake the unblinding).

In case of SUSARs the following safety issues require expedited reporting:

- Single case reports of an expected serious adverse reaction with an unexpected outcome (*e.g.*: a fatal outcome)
- An increase in the rate of occurrence of an expected serious adverse reaction, which is judged to be clinically important
- Post-study SUSARs that occur after the patient has completed a clinical trial and are notified by the investigator to the sponsor should be reported to the MHRA indefinitely.

Data Elements for SUSAR Report

1. ***Clinical trial identification***
   - Clinical trial identification (EudraCT number, if applicable or the sponsor's trial protocol number).
2. ***Subject's details***
   - Sponsor's subject identification number,
   - Initials, if applicable,
   - Gender,
   - Age and/or date of birth,
   - Weight,
   - Height,
3. ***Suspected investigational medicinal product(s)***
   - Name of the investigational medicinal product or brand name as reported,
   - International non-proprietary name (INN),
   - Batch number,
   - Indication(s) for which suspect investigational medicinal product was prescribed or tested,
   - Dosage form and strength,
   - Daily dose and regimen (specify units *e.g.* mg, ml, mg/kg),
   - Route of administration,
   - Starting date and time of day,
   - Stopping date and time, or duration of treatment

- Unblinding: yes/no/not applicable; results
- Investigators' causality assessment
- Sponsors' causality assessment
- Comments– if relevant (*e.g:* causality assessment if the sponsor disagrees with the reporter; concomitant medications suspected to play role in the reactions directly or by interaction; indication treated with suspect drug(s).

4. ***Other treatment(s)***
   - For concomitant medicinal products (including non prescription/ OTC medicinal products) and non-medicinal product therapies provide the same information as listed above for the suspected investigational medicinal product.
5. ***Details of suspected adverse drug reaction(s)***
   - Full description of reaction(s) including body site and severity, as well as the criterion (or criteria) for regarding the report as serious should be given. In addition to a description of the reported signs and symptoms, whenever possible attempts should be made to establish a specific diagnosis for the reaction,
   - Reaction(s) in MedDRA terminology1 (lowest level term)
   - Start date (and time) of onset of the reaction,
   - Stop date (and time) or duration of the reaction,
   - De-challenge and re-challenge information,
   - Setting (*e.g*. hospital, out-patient clinic, home, nursing home),
   - *Outcome: information on recovery and any sequelae;* what specific tests and/or treatment may have been required and their results; for a fatal outcome, cause of death and a comment on its possible relationship to the suspected reaction should be provided. Any autopsy or other post-mortem findings (including a coroner's report) should also be provided when available,
   - *Other information:* anything relevant to facilitate assessment of the case, such as medical history including allergy, drug or alcohol abuse, family history, findings from special investigations.
6. ***Details on reporter of event / suspected adverse reactions***
   - Name,
   - Address,

- Telephone number,
- Profession (speciality).

7. ***Administrative and sponsor details***
   - Date of this report,
   - Source of report: from a clinical trial (provide details if not in Eudract 1, from the literature (provide copy), spontaneous, other,
   - Date event report was first received by sponsor,
   - Country in which reaction occurred,
   - Type of report filed to authorities: initial or follow-up (first, second, etc),
   - Name and address of sponsor/manufacturer/company,
   - Name, address, telephone number and fax number of contact person in reporting sponsor,
   - Identifying regulatory code or number for marketing authorisation dossier or clinical investigation process for the suspected product (for example IND number, NDA number),
   - Case reference number (sponsor's/manufacturer's identification number for the case) (this number must be the same for the initial and follow-up reports on the same case).

There is expedited reporting essential in case of SUSARS. The Regulations have set time limits for expedited reporting. In case of fatal or life threatening SUSARs, it is not later than 7 calendar days after the sponsor has information that the case reported fulfils the criteria for a fatal or life-threatening SUSAR, with any follow up information to be reported within a further 8 calendar days. And in case of all other SUSARs, it should be not later than 15 calendar days after the sponsor has information that the case fulfilled the criteria for a SUSAR.

Thus PSURs and SUSARs were initiatives taken to harmonsie the process for safety reports submission to regulatory authorities. As the world started noticing the requirement of more stringent pharmacovigilance studies for the betterment of the society, many more changes took place and there was an addendum to the PSUR after CIOMS II initiative which was reflected in CIOMS V. Requirements such as confidentiality of proprietary information, risk management programs and benefit-risk analysis were included to strengthen the Pharmacovigilance system further.

10

Drug Safety of Biopharmaceuticals and Biosimilars

Biopharmaceuticals amount to several billion dollar sales in the United States. This huge sales is majorly contributed by the four main biopharmaceuticals, *viz*: insulin, growth hormone (GH), and granulocyte colony stimulating factor (G-CSF). The progress over the last quarter of a century made in the area of recombinant DNA technology have lead to the large-scale manufacture of biologically-engineered proteins within living cells. Biopharmaceuticals' patents which have expired or are in the verge of expiring (*e.g.*: Humulin®, Intron A®, Procrit®/Eprex®, and Neupogen®) is taken up for production of a similar product known as biosimilars. Before plunging into the pharmacovigilance of biosimilars, it is very important to understand the specifics of how Biosimilars are different from small molecules. This is precisely the reason why Biosimilars' pharmacovigilance studies have been carved out in a different chapter. Bio-similars also known as biogenerics or follow on biologics, due to their unique and different characteristics from one another also carry their own risks unlike small molecules. This is largely due to the fact that biopharmaceuticals are manufactured in living cells unlike small molecules which are synthesized in a chemical manner. Thus despite of mimicking the process of synthesis to the innovator in case of biosimilars, the two products will not be the same.

Biosimilars are defined by the European Medicines Agency (EMEA) as biopharmaceuticals claimed to be similar to a reference medicinal product based on the demonstration of the similar nature of the two products, in terms of quality, safety and efficacy. When the safety and efficacy of the reference product and biosimilar are comparable, the biosimilar product is thereby approved on the basis of a submitted ANDA. Few pharmaceutical companies have taken the plunge of manufacturing a biosimilar (as discussed above) because of the patent expiration of some innovator products like growth hormones, granulocyte colony stimulating factors, and erythropoietin. Thus to get a biosimilar product approved pharmaceutical company needs to show a comparative study of the safety and efficacy of the reference and the biogeneric. The approval of a biosimilar recombinant derived growth hormone Valtropin of a reference product Humatrope was an interesting case study indeed. It was agreed in this particular case that when therapeutic comparability between the reference and biogeneric product is proved in one particular indication, the comparability is automatically set for other indications as observed in the reference product. This means that the extrapolation of the therapeutic compatibility can be performed in other indications when it is proven for one indication. In this case a comparative double-blind phase III study of the reference product Humatrope and Valtropin was conducted. It was agreed in this comparative study that the indication 'Children with growth hormone deficiency' could be extrapolated to all indications for which the reference product Humatrope had already been approved. But this kind of an extrapolation can be a serious limitation with regards to the safety profile. As discussed, unlike small molecules, biopharmaceuticals have a very complicated and tedious process of manufacture in living cells and it involves several steps. Small changes in the production and purification process can have major implications on the safety profile of the biopharmaceutical, which is also the case in the production process after the biopharmaceutical has already been marketed. It has to be borne in mind that unlike small molecules, it is very difficult or practically impossible for manufacturer of biosimilars to replicate the protein product step by step in an exact manner which in turn, might have an impact on the safety profile. The characteristics of biopharmaceuticals are closely related to the production process, which is very difficult to duplicate. As manufacturing protocols are quite often the proprietary knowledge of the originator company, it is impossible for a biosimilar's manufacturer to duplicate the process. This may therefore lead to structural differences in the biosimilar molecule being produced. Like for instance, the three dimensional structure of the protein and the glycosylation profile may not be replicated in a accurate manner thus leading to dissimilarities between the reference product and the biosimilar. This means the product obtained at the end of the synthetic process may have a different set of characteristics as compared to the reference and hence can also influence the safety profile of the biogeneric. This means despite the fact that biosimilar and reference product can show similar efficacy, the biosimilar may exhibit different safety profile with regards to nature, seriousness or incidence of adverse reactions. Thus clinical safety and the benefit-risk assessment of the biogenerics must be monitored closely on ongoing basis during the post approval phase.

Thus, summing it all up, the reasons for concern with regards to the biosimilar for manufacturers, regulatory bodies, patients, include:

1. Testing for similarity and comparability of the biosimilars with the originator products.
2. Guidelines for long-term pharmacovigilance programmes and
3. Assessment of potential complications arising from both short and long-term use.

The most significant safety concern pertaining to biopharmaceuticals including biosimilars is immunogenicity. All biopharmaceuticals are biologically active molecules derived from living cells, and have all probability to stir an immune response. Several assays based on conformational dependent antibodies are used for predictions of immunoreactivity. The complexities in the manufacturing process of the biogeneric which is distinct from the reference biological, can alter the immunogenicity profile of the biosimilar compared to the reference product. Immunogenicity, including lack of efficacy, is therefore an important (potential) safety problem, which should specifically be taken into account. The immunogenicity which leads to lack of efficacy is a safety issue and needs special focus and mention whilst submitting a PSUR. Biopharmaceuticals run the risk of immunogenicity in patients and although immune responses to biopharmaceuticals are not frequently associated with adverse events, immunogenicity can cause serious safety problems. Thus an extrapolation from preclinical data to clinical data in humans is a serious limitation in case of biopharmaceuticals.

Immunogenecity can occur due to the following reasons:

1. Impurities of the end product;
2. Structural modifications due to the different manufacturing process;
3. Formation of aggregates;
4. Nature of the protein (endogenous/non-endogenous) and/or
5. Storage conditions
6. Route of administration of the biopharmaceutical
7. Genetic background
8. HLA expression of the patient
9. Type of disease
10. Patients' immune status

By adopting adequate quality control measures during the manufacturing process and stringent testing of the medicinal product during its development, the risk of immunogenicity can be reduced and safe products of consistent quality can be obtained. Binding of neutralizing antibodies to the biopharmaceutical product can neutralize biological activity of the product and also effect biological elimination. Due to this the clearance is decreased and the half life elimination of the product is prolonged. Besides, inhibitory antibodies to interferon (IFN) beta, a product used in the treatment of multiple sclerosis caused many patients to withdraw from treatment. Inhibitory antibodies to PEGylated megakaryocyte growth and development factor (MDGF) caused thrombocytopenia in healthy volunteers enrolled for clinical trials.

There are series of instances wherein reactions were caused by a biopharmaceutical product due to species to species variation:

1. Biopharmaceutical formulation recombinant human epoetin (Eprex) when given to patients triggered the incidence of pure red cell aplasia (PRCA) which is caused by antibodies.
2. Incidence of thrombocytopenia after treatment with recombinant thrombopoetin due to neutralizing antibodies.
3. Cytokine storm in the TeGenero phase I trial, in which healthy volunteers were treated with a monoclonal antibody for the first time.
4. Human proteins leading to immunogenicity in animals.

Eprex® (epoetin alfa) is a biopharmaceutical used in treatment of anaemia, secondary to chronic kidney disease to help produce adequate amounts of endogenous erythropoietin. We shall now see, how minor changes during the manufacture of the product leads to safety issues. Minor changes during the manufacturing process led to production of neutralising antibodies to the injected epoetin as well as endogenous erythropoietin making the bone marrow aplastic for erythropoietic progenitor cells (PRCA).

The various *in-vitro* tests are done for comparison of structural aspects, primary aminoacid sequence, chargé and hydrophobic properties of Biosimilars with the reference biologicals. Nuclear Magnetic Resonance Spectroscopy (NMR) or MS is used for determination of higher order structure. *In-vitro* results cannot be extrapolated to *in-vivo* biological activity although they may be similar in terms of structure and size to the reference product. Also pre-clinical studies is not a solution to predict the biological activity *in-vivo* in humans; as only a very handful of the data obtained from animal models can actually be extrapolated as such in humans. Further clinical trials also pose their own constraints like inefficiency in detecting the sporadic iatrogenic reactions.

It needs to be understood therefore as discussed above, that since the product obtained as a biogenéric or biosimilar has different characteristics as compared to the innovator, the safety profiles also accordingly vary. Thus another point of significance is that, since safety profile is anticipated to be different in case of a biosimilar, the safety studies become all the more important in such a scenario. This is because, due to obvious constraints of conducting randomized clinical trials, an abbreviated dossier is thus submitted for obtainment of a marketing license of a biosimilar. Thus from a regulatory standpoint, there is a conscious effort needed to bring about changes and improvement in the pharmacovigilance of biosimilars.

The EMEA and the Committee for Human Medicinal Products (CHMP) are authorities which are in the process of framing stringent guidelines for biosimilars. This is required to constantly and vigorously monitor the safety, activity and efficacy of the biosimilars. The guidelines would focus on non-clinical and clinical issues of biosimilars which would include manufacturing processes, quality control and guidelines specific to different classes of biosimilars such as recombinant human GH, insulin, erythropoietin and G-CSF.

New, rare and/or serious ADRs can be detected by spontaneous reporting of adverse drug reactions (ADRs) in case of biopharmaceuticals. As discussed earlier, that it is not possible to produce an exact replica or identical to the reference product and thus the characteristics and safety profile of the biosimilar will be different from the reference product. So to aid in identifying the differences between safety profile of the reference product and biosimilar, collection of ADR reports *via* spontaneous reporting will be beneficial. Spontaneous reporting and submission of Periodic Safety Update Reports (PSURs) to the regulatory authorities, is obligatory for all medicinal products marketed in the European Union.

Under reporting, missing exposure data and difficulties in assessing the causality between the ADR and the drug of interest are some of the common setbacks associated with spontaneous reporting. However with biopharmaceuticals there are some of some interesting situations which can be a limitation as such.

1. ***Switching over to other biopharmaceuticals of the same active susbstance while one therapy is already going on:*** Is not appreciable and can be a hindrance while utilizing the spontaneous reporting facility to its full potential. This is because when an ADR occurs, it would be difficult to identify the real culprit or suspect drug which actually caused the ADR. The situation becomes even worse when the ADR occur with a long latency period; *i.e.* the time between the exposure of the drug and the occurence of the ADR is high. Thus the causality assessment becomes rather tough in such a scenario. Hence switching between biopharmaceuticals must be strictly prohibited.

   For instance, the analysis of lymphoma risks in patients suffering from inflammatory bowel disease and treated with infliximab, which was confounded by concomitant use of other immunosuppressive agents.

2. According to the current naming system by World Health Organization (WHO), biosimilars receive the same international nonproprietary name (INN) as the reference product. An identifiable suspect drug is very important as per the norms of

pharmacovigilance studies. Because of the naming system of WHO, even a biosimilar receives the same INN as that of the reference product. Thus it can be misleading if the ADR is caused due to a biosimilar and not due to the innovator product. Hence it is very important to firstly distinguish between the biosimilar and the reference product. An identifiable name ought to be given to the biosimilar which is different from the INN. Thus biological should always be commercialized with a brand name or the INN plus the manufacturers' name.

3. Batch number and production date are very significant informations to identification of biopharmaceuticals and thus recording of these information should be a must while spontaneous reporting of ADR.
4. Information pertaining to the indication for which the biosimilar is used needs to be recorded as well, and the ADR needs to be pooled together under a specific indication banner. This is essential in case of biosimilar for which a clinical trial has not been conducted.

After the product gets marketing authorization, once the product is on market, the manufacturer has to submit PSURs (which provide an update on worldwide safety aspect of the product) to the regulatory authority. Also alternative biopharmaceuticals containing the same active substance, needs a mention in the PSUR. To avoid repetitive actions being taken on a biopharmaceutical containing the same active susbstance, the PSUR of the biosimilar mentioning alerts of safety signal needs to be checked meticulously.

Risk Management Plan

Risk management plan includes scientifically based methodologies to identify, assess, communicate and minimize risk throughout a drugs' life cycle so as to establish a favorable benefit-risk profile in patients. It has been European Unions' initiative that manufacturers who deal with either new substance or a biosimilar should submit a Risk Management plan. This should be done taking into consideration the Benefit-Risk ratio as explained in previous chapter. And accordingly a plan chalking out strategies to mitigate the risk needs to be prepared and submitted as a part of marketing application. This is known as a risk management plan. The manufacturers' are obliged to do this since Nov 2005.

Risks are classified into three different types for convenience:

1. Identified risks (there is a clear causal association between the drug and the ADR),
2. Potential risks (there is no clear association between the drug and the ADR but there might be an association, *e.g*. an ADR which is expected based on the pharmacology but was not seen in the pre-registration trials), and
3. Missing information including populations not studied in the pre-authorization phase.

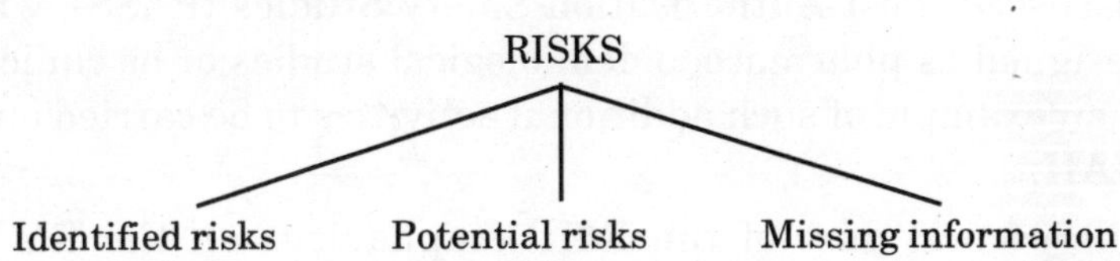

Fig. 3: Types of risks

The objective of a RMP is proactive risk management. This is necessary to take control of any risks possible due to the medicinal product and try preventing or mitigating it by providing logical solutions. The RMP consists of two parts.

1. The first part of the RMP includes Safety specification and Pharmacovigilance plan which are discussed in detail below.

   Safety specification: Must recapitulate the results and limitations of the performed pre-registration studies. The safety specification summarizes the safety profile of the drug at a particular point in time. As discussed above, risks are classified at three different levels; identified risks wherein there is a clear causal association between the drug and the ADR), potential risks where there is no clear association between the drug and the ADR but there might be an association, *e.g*. an ADR which is expected based on the pharmacology but was not seen in the pre-registration trials, and missing information including populations not studied in the pre-authorization phase.

Pharmacovigilance plan: This plan is necessary so that the marketing authorization holder analyses thoroughly the details regarding the medicinal product and derive if there is any probable safety issue or risk due to the medicinal product. The product may not obviously seem to have any safety concern, but there may be a possibility which might later show up. So to avoid this and to double check the additional activities are carried out. It is needed to suggest action to further study and quantify potential safety concerns. It should contain the additional activities a marketing authorization holder (MAH) will perform to recognize and compute safety concerns. Apart from the mandatory routine pharmacovigilance activities, as mentioned above, the additional pharmacovigilance activities that will be carried out needs to be discussed. Post-Authorisation Safety Studies (PASS), which are designed as pharmacoepidemiological studies or as clinical trials is an example of such additional activities to be carried out by the MAH.

2. The second part of the RMP emphasizes on the RMP being complete to the core. It has to be noted that safety specification should not be formulated only taking into consideration the already available data from pre-registration trials, but along side the safety alerts that arise also from the reference product and other biopharmaceuticals which essentially contain the same active substance must be included also. Further the need for additional activities with regards the biosimilar must be included along with any information available regarding the reference product must be incorporated. The MAH of the biosimilar must also participate in the ongoing studies of the reference product. Now the need for additional activities spurs from the fact that some indications for which a biosimilar might be used, its trials may not be conducted in the pre-registration phase. Again the additional activities are very essential because the safety profiles may not be the same for two different indications of the same biosimilar product. Besides this, the biosimilar may be used for a certain offlabel activity for which the reference product might be actually approved. And because of the very complex nature of a biopharmaceutical and in addition the complex process of manufacture of the product, the biosimilar and the reference are not identical. Hence the safety

profiles are different, due to which an offlabel use may be very risky. Thus collection of the offlabel use data of the biosimilar is very essential. In addition, immunogenicity, including lack of efficacy, and (very) rare and serious ADRs should particularly be tackled in the RMP and the need for additional pharmacovigilance activities should be clearly evaluated. Thus in a nut shell the second part of the RMP summarizes the risk minimization activities that is generally carried out and assesses the need for additional risk minimization activities.

Some Examples

The biosimilar product EpoetinalfaHexal did not show PRCA but was seen in the reference product, Eprex. Thus the RMP should conduct additional activities for confirming the safety profile of EpoetinalfaHexal and tests to identify PRCA with biosimilar needs to be done.

Further EpoetinalfaHexal is not approved for subcutaneous administration in patients with anemia associated with renal failure. Thus, ideally a market survey needs to be done to evaluate the safety profile of off-label subcutaneous use in renal anaemia patients, as laid down in the RMP.

The RMP should also propose methods for better identification of products during the normal regular studies and also whilst the additional activities undertaken. Thus there should be no scope for confusion between the biosimilar and the reference product. Since both are given the same INN by the WHO, the identification can be a problem and hence the RMP should suggest methods to improve the identifiability of the medicinal product.

Production of biopharmaceutical, reference product is a proprietary knowledge of MAH and involves a complicated process including multiple steps. Thus the biosimilar whilst it's manufacturing process cannot be identical and leads to the formation of a similar but not a replica of the reference product. Owing to this, the safety profiles of the reference product and biosimilar are quite different. Thus it is very necessary that the data regarding the safety concerns related to the biosimilar be collected promptly by spontaneous reporting.

Therefore the following points need to be considered while assessing the safety of a biosimilar:

1. Immunogenicity including lack of efficacy can be a serious issue.
2. Identifiability of the suspect drug, *i.e.* biosimilar this is because WHO gives an INN for both the biopharmaceutical reference product and the biosimilar.
3. The safety profile assessment of biosimilar is very essential because the safety of the biosimilar is very different from the reference product.
4. Since the therapeutic comparability done between the reference product and biosimilar is extrapolated from one indication to other indications of a biosimilar, this can be a serious issue while using the biosimilar in real life by patients. Hence the safety profiles must be thoroughly assessed for other indications to for a biosimilar product.

11

Pharmacoepidemiology

Pharmacoepidemiology is the study of the use of and effects of, drugs in large numbers of people. As the term implies, this form of enquiry uses the methods of epidemiology; it is concerned with all aspects of the benefit-risk ratio of drugs in populations. Pharmacovigilance is a branch of pharmacoepidemiology but is restricted to the study, on an epidemiological scale, of drug events or adverse reactions. 'Events', in this context, are happenings recorded in the patient's notes during a period of drug monitoring; they may be because of the disease for which the drug is being given, some other intercurrent disease or infection, an adverse reaction to the drug being monitored or the activity of a drug being given concomitantly. They can also be because of drug–drug interactions. Public health surveillance methods are used to identify new signals of possible ADRs. Studies in pharmacoepidemiology are intended to be either 'hypothesis generating' or 'hypothesis-testing' or to share these objectives. Hypothesis-generating studies, with a recently marketed drug, aim to detect unexpected ADRs; hypothesis-testing studies aim to prove whether any suspicions that may have been raised are justified.

Popular brand names like Vioxx being withdrawn from the market led to big pharmaceutical companies suffering shocks to profitability and share price erosion. An ounce of prevention in the form of early detection of AE signals and accurate risk assessment in such an unpredictable ambiance can forestall profound business and consumer losses. Thus in 2005, US FDA issued three safety guidances, viz: premarketing risk assessment, Use of RMPs, Good Pharmacovigilance practices and pharmacoepidemiological assessment.

FDA recognizes that there are a variety of methods for investigating a safety signal. Signals warranting supplementary investigation can be further evaluated through carefully designed nonrandomized observational studies of the product's use in the "real world" and randomized trials. The Premarketing Guidance discusses a number of types of randomized trials, including the large simple safety study, which is a risk assessment method that could be used either pre- or post-approval.

Albeit there are many types of non-randomized observational studies, the three main are:

1. Pharmacoepidemiologic studies,
2. Registries, and
3. Surveys.

FDA encourages sponsors to consider all methods to evaluate a particular safety signal and recommends that sponsors choose the method best suited to the particular signal and research question of interest.

Pharmacoepidemiology is the scientific backbone of therapeutic risk management-the process of assessing a product's benefits and risks, and developing, implementing, and evaluating strategies to enhance the overall balance of such benefits and risks. Pharmacoepidemiologic (PE) studies can be of various types which include cohort (prospective or retrospective), case-control, nested case-control, case-crossover, or other models. The results of such studies may be used to characterize one or more safety signals associated with a product, or may examine the natural history of a disease or drug utilization patterns. PE study being designed to assess the risk attributed to a drug exposure has a protocol and control group and tests prespecified hypothesis. Both relative risk of an outcome associated with a product, and some (*e.g.*, cohort studies) and incidence rate pertaining to risk for an adverse event can be estimated from PE studies. Sponsors can initiate pharmacoepidemiologic studies at any time. They are sometimes started at the time of initial marketing, based on questions that remain after review of the premarketing data. More often, however, they are initiated when a safety signal has been identified after approval. For uncommon or delayed adverse events, pharmacoepidemiologic studies may be the only practical choice for evaluation, even though they can be limited by low statistical power. Finally, there may also be occasions when a pharmacoepidemiologic study is initiated prior to marketing (*e.g.*, to study the natural history of disease or patterns of product use, or to estimate background rates for adverse events). Clinical trials are impractical in almost all cases when the event rates of concern are less common than 1:2000–3000 (an exception may be larger trials conducted for some vaccines, which could move the threshold to 1:10,000).

Thus pharmacoepidemiological studies must ensure that:

1. Spontaneous reports of suspected adverse reactions must be used to the full potential *i.e.* considering all the implications of the suspect drug at hand to have caused the reaction, the reasons and mechanisms which probably led to the reaction without missing any signal.
2. The other sources of information which are available shall be used to interpret the data rapidly within timelines. This means that instead of waiting for too long to confirm and reconfirm till a specific data arrives, many lives, lot of money, and time can be saved by utilizing the information at hand.
3. Solutions to existing problems due to adverse drug reactions must be given with a thorough study of data in hand. The motto should be save lives as much as possible and as many as possible.

It may also be complicated to use clinical trials: (1) to evaluate a safety signal associated with constant exposure to a product, exposure in populations with co-morbid conditions, or taking multiple concomitant medications, or (2) to identify certain risk factors for a particular adverse event. On the other hand, for evaluation of more common events, which are seen relatively often in untreated patients, clinical trials may be preferable to observational studies. When the relative risk to exposed patients is high, the issues pertaining to pharmacoepidemiologic studies such as, being observational in nature, subject to confounding, effect modification, and other preconceived notions, can be surmounted. Otherwise in the *vice versa* scenario, the results of these types of studies become more difficult to interpret than the results of clinical trials. Benefit-risk considerations, *viz.*, seriousness of the disease being treated, nature and frequency of the safety signal under evaluation are diverse for different products and hence generally become impossible to delineate a universal set of criteria. For this reason pharmacoepidemiologic study decisions and study initiation should be made on a case-by-case basis. When an important adverse event–product association leads to questions on the product's benefit-risk balance, then the sponsors needs to take a decision whether the particular signal should be addressed with one or more pharmacoepidemiologic studies. Objectives of the study and expected frequency of the events of interest are the two main criteria to be considered while formulating the design and size of the proposed study. When performing a pharmacoepidemiologic study, the investigators must seek to minimize bias and to account for possible confounding. Confounding by indication is one example of an important concern in performing a pharmacoepidemiologic study. Conflicting results arise due to bias, confounding, or effect modification, in pharmacoepidemiologic studies even if the hypothesis is same. PE studies being observational, it is almost always prudent to conduct more than one study, in more than one environment and even use different designs. This often gives a reassurance that the observed results are robust.

A protocol for a pharmacoepidemiologic study generally includes:

1. Clearly specified study objectives;
2. A critical review of the literature; and
3. A detailed description of the research methods, including:
   - the population to be studied;
   - the case definitions to be used;
   - the data sources to be used (including a rationale for data sources);
   - the projected study size and statistical power calculations; and
   - the methods for data collection, management, and analysis.

Depending on the kind of pharmacoepidemiologic study planned, there are an array of data sources that may be used, ranging from the prospective collection of data to the use of existing data, such as data from previously conducted clinical trials or large databases. In recent years, a number of pharmacoepidemiologic studies have been conducted in automated claims databases which permit retrieval of records on product exposure and patient outcomes. In addition, recently, comprehensive electronic medical record databases have also been used for studying drug safety issues.

Depending on study objectives, factors that may affect the choice of databases include the following:

1. Demographic characteristics of patients enrolled in the health plans (*e.g.*, age, geographic location);
2. Turnover rate of patients in the health plans;
3. Plan coverage of the medications of interest;
4. Size and characteristics of the exposed population available for study;
5. Availability of the outcomes of interest;
6. Ability to identify conditions of interest using standard medical coding systems (*e.g.*, International Classification of Diseases (ICD-9)), procedure codes or prescriptions that could be used as markers.
7. Access to medical records; and
8. Access to patients for data not captured electronically.

Diagnostic findings need to be validated through a detailed review of at least a sample of medical records. If the validation of the specific outcome or exposure of interest using the proposed database has been previously reported, then it is recommended that the literature supporting the validity of the proposed study be submitted for review.

Wherever further investigation and analysis is warranted, like in case of an excess of adverse events or safety signal, it is important to put the signal into context. For this reason, calculations such as incidence rate, *i.e.* the rate at which new cases of adverse events occur in the product-exposed population are the characteristic of pharmacoepidemiologic risk assessment. In pharmacoepidemiologic studies, the numerator (number of new cases) and denominator (number of exposed patients and time of exposure or, if known, time at risk) may be readily ascertainable. In contrast, for spontaneously reported events, it is not possible to identify all cases because of under-reporting, and the size of the population at risk is at best a guesstimate.

Limitations in national denominator estimates arise because:

1. Accurate national estimates of the number of patients exposed to a medical product and their duration of exposure may not be available;
2. It may be difficult to exclude patients who are not at risk for an event, for example, because their exposure is too brief or their dose is too low;
3. A product may be used in different populations for different indications, but used estimates are not available for the specific population of interest. Although we recognize these limitations, we recommend that sponsors calculate crude adverse event reporting rates as a valuable step in the investigation and assessment of adverse events. Reporting rates may be calculated by using the total number of spontaneously reported cases in the numerator and estimates of national patient exposure to product in the denominator. It is recommended that whenever possible, the number of patients or person time exposed to the product nationwide be the estimated denominator for a reporting rate. Other replacements for exposure, such as numbers of prescriptions or kilograms of product sold, only be used when patient-level approximations are unavailable. A detailed explanation of the rationale for selection of a denominator and a method of estimation needs to be submitted. Comparisons of reporting rates and their temporal trends can be valuable, particularly across similar products or across different product classes prescribed for the same indication. However, inherent uncertainties in the numerator and denominator used are certain limitations with regard to their interpretation. As a result, it is suggested that a comparison of two or more reporting rates be viewed with extreme caution and generally considered exploratory or hypothesis generating. For absolute or comparative purposes, it is helpful to have an estimate of the background rate of occurrence for the event being evaluated in the general population, since reporting rates by no means can be considered as incidence rates. This is also true in case of subpopulation with characteristics similar to that of the exposed population (*e.g.*, premenopausal women, diabetics).

These background rates can be derived from:

1. national health statistics,
2. published medical literature, or
3. ad hoc studies, particularly of subpopulations, using large automated databases or ongoing epidemiologic investigations with primary data collection.

Comparisons of incidence rates or reporting rates to background rate estimates take into account potential differences in the data sources, diagnostic criteria, and duration of time at risk. While the extent of under-reporting is unknown, it is usually assumed to be substantial and may vary according to the type of product, seriousness of the event, population using the product, and other factors. As a result, a reporting rate higher than the background rate may, in some cases, be a strong indicator that the true incidence rate is sufficiently high to be of concern. However, many other factors affect the reporting of product-related adverse events (*e.g.*, publicity, newness of product to the market) and these factors should be considered when interpreting a high reporting rate. Also, because of under-reporting, the fact that a reporting rate is less than the background rate does not necessarily show that the product is not associated with an increased risk of an adverse event.

The safety and effectiveness of drugs information generated from pharmacoepidemiologic studies can yield generate significant information for pharmacoeconomic evaluation a specific drug therapy. The natural progression of disease comorbidities and treatment can enable assessing variables that may have pharmacoeconomic implications with respect to cost of illness and quality of life.

12

Pharmacoeconomics

Pharmacoeconomics has been defined as the "description and analysis of costs of drug therapy to health care systems and society. In other words the cost-benefit or cost-consequences estimates are done. Pharmacoeconomic (PE) research identifies, measures, and compares the resources consumed and consequences which include economic, humanistic and clinical results of pharmaceutical goods (products) and services. Thus cost-effectiveness, cost-minimization, cost-benefits, cost-of-illness, cost-utility, cost-consequences, decision analysis, quality of life and other humanistic assessment are all necessary as research methods do not only assess outcomes but also to put it in perspective of other health expenditures. These methods have been derived from various areas like: economics, epidemiology, social sciences, medicine and pharmacy. Both the fiscal parameter and delivery with respect to healthcare system will be adequately handled because of pharmacoeconomic analysis. The pharmacoeconomic analysis thus done in the above ways will help in the results being practically applied by practitioners in therapeutic decision making which shall positively influence patient outcomes. This would play a vey important role in situations wherein the patient who needs emergency care is not able to utilize the facility just because he cannot afford the same. This ofcourse is not limited to emergency care alone and extends to various other circumstances like medical care needed in case of diseases such as cancer, malaria etc and also in some milder situations which may need long term care. Pharmacoeconomic evaluation is an analytical tool used with increasing frequency to assist decision making in the financing and management of pharmaceutical products in the health care system or national health insurance programs of an individual country. So it is very evident as to how pharmacoeconomics can play a very significant role in healthcare and thus awareness and knowledge regarding the same becomes quintessential.

Pharmacoeconomics may thus help in imparting quality patient care by addressing the following points:

- The best drug for a particular patient
- The best drug for a particular disease
- The best drug for a pharmaceutical manufacturer to develop
- The drug delivery system that would be the best for the hospital
- The drugs to be included in the hospital formulary
- The cost pertaining to a drug by which a quality year of life was given to the patient.
- A drug therapy decision which would improve the quality of life of a patient.
- Patient outcomes for various treatment modalities

From the above mentioned points, we can say that pharamacoeconomics behaves in a multidimensional pattern catering to the needs of the patient, the interest of the manufacturers, hospitals and society at large. Thus pharmacoeconomics analysis uses tools for examining the impact or outcomes of drug therapies and other related medical interventions.

Assessing cost-effectiveness analyses and the future of health technology assessment (HTA) in healthcare decision are major parameters as far as pharmacoeconomics is concerned.

Why is Pharmacoeconomics Significant for Developing Countries?

The practical utility of pharmacoeconomics depends on the context in which it is being applied. Since this complex science is used in both financing and management of pharmaceutical products in the health care system, it can be referred to as a pillar based on which the pharmaceutical industry stands. The full potential of pharmacoeconomics needs to be utilized in making appropriate heathcare decisions. This goes on to say that the jurisdiction wherein the pharmacoeconomic techniques would be applied needs to be considered and high importance needs to be given to the same. If the local health system is such that, the economic techniques will not be workable, then planning and developing makes no sense? Or else the option is to convince the local health systems and public regarding these techniques for their own benefits. The perception of public towards pharmacoeconomics, Health and pharmaceutical indicators and evidence-based pharmacy-system research could serve as components for formulary development of a developing country. Also awareness of Pharmacoeconomics in developing Countries needs to be generated.

Having said this, the country's expenditure on pharmaceutical and healthcare needs has to be thoroughly understood. Is the country meticulously analyzing the health care needs of the people at large, or is it an underestimate of what actually needs to be done. Are the entire needs of healthcare per se catered to, considering the urban, semi-urban, and rural areas of the nation? Thus assessing the pharmaceutical situation of a country requires pharmaceutical sector assessment, including whether people have access to safe, effective and affordable essential medicines of acceptable quality. A link to compare the pharmacy services and treatment options is pharmacoeconomics. So when it comes to peple from various social and economic backgrounds, the treatment options must be ready but at the same time giving them the best possible quality medical care. Hence, the utility of pharmacoeconomics for selecting drugs for national medicines formularies depends on various factors, including health system design and performance, the pharmaceutical situation and the country's expenditure on pharmaceuticals. It is thus very evident from the discussion above that an appropriate pricing policy should be the first step towards the growth of pharmacoeconomics in a country. So depending on a country's economic growth and pharmaceutical or heathcare system development, either innovator or generic medicines could be used as first line strategies. Like for instance, in a developed country use of innovator could be rather easy but at the same time for a developing country or under developed country generics would form a part of the first line strategies. For many low-income countries there is no necessity to use complex 'cost utility or cost-effectiveness techniques' for selecting drugs for a national formulary. In a nutshell, whatever may be the economic background of a country, the essence of phamracoeconomics will be to utilize the available healthcare resources to its full potential and at an affordable range. If the available heathcare resources are priced high, then the solution would be to take giant strides towards developing a formlation which shall be available at a reasonable price. For example: Taiwan, the Philippines, South Korea, Thailand and Malaysia are at different levels of 'health system development', but in all these countries "pharmacoeconomics has been or will be increasingly used. WHO medicines policy framework, rational pricing policies and the use of generic medicines as first-line strategies is more workable for the Philippines, Malaysia and Thailand.

As discussed earlier, the applicability of pharmacoeconomics is possible only if the the country is able to work it out in a full fledged manner. With Health Technology assessment progressing at different velocities in various countries, it is evident that dependent on the individual health systems the applicability of pharmacoeconomics shall be based. Depending on, the socioeconomic status of a given country, pharmaceutical reforms, and the advancement and maturity of independent health systems we shall categorize countries into three groups, viz: Group 1, Group 2 and Group 3. For explaining and understanding the essence of pharmacoeconomics better we taken into consideration the following grouping.

GROUP 1: SOUTH KOREA AND TAIWAN

Pharmacy system research is an indispensable part of the national health policy of a country. Pharmacy system research comprises of research related to drug distribution, drug regulation, drug selection, procurement, pricing, generic medicines, and access and affordability of medicines. Advanced pharmaceutical systems and regulatory structures pertaining to pharmaceuticals are in place for both these countries. The gross national income, pharmaceuticals related expenditure, health system performance and appropriate pharmacovigilance system in place are all indicators of such a progress in these countries. They have been part of major pharmaceutical policy reforms and handled major issues such as differentiating the role of pharmacists and doctors in prescribing to patients. The Centre for Drug

Evaluation (CDE) in Taiwan is iconic of an advanced pharmaceutical system and would encourage pharmacoeconomic models to support reasonable medical expenditures. CDE takes care of regulatory assessments of new drugs, the dossiers pertaining to the product and also advises health department of Taiwan. Health Insurance Review Agency (HIRA) of South Korea prepares economic data in accordance to the guidelines to submit the same for pricing etc. To establish a national agency in South Korea like NICE of UK is on the way.

GROUP 2: IRAN, MALAYSIA

Medicines, Affordability and Medicine Reimbursement

An appropriate pharmacoeconomics model in these countries can play a vital role because certain issues including pricing are still complex and unfair. Not going too far, to understand this, lets take the instance of Malaysian drug prices. The branded and generic drugs were found to be 16 and 6-old higher than international reference prices (IRPs), respectively. Thus a quick measure needs to be taken here. WHO and Health Action International (HAI) have set right a standard method to calculate such pricing ratios of pharmaceuticals in developing countries. The ratio indicates if the price is low or high. If this ratio is <1 for public sector data (government hospitals, clinics, etc.) and <2 for private sector data (private pharmacies, medical stores), then the prices are considered reasonable. Iran has the systems in place and is indicative of a good pricing system for generics which is provided at affordable range. This was also confirmed by a WHO/HAI analysis. About 90% of population has access to safe and effective medicines which is a huge number indeed. But some of the innovators were an average of 3- to 7-fold higher than the price of generic equivalents. A 6- to 9-fold higher than the IRPs, were found in case of Digoxin, metformin and carbamazepine. Iran has a good pharmacy-system research in place, and has a good understanding of pharmacoeconomics

GROUP 3: INDONESIA, PAKISTAN, THAILAND AND THE PHILIPPINES,

Indonesia, Pakistan, Thailand and the Philippines are those countries whose drug regulatory authorities need strengthening. They rank from

99 to 124 of 191 countries in terms of health system performance according to disability-adjusted life-expectancy. ALos that the income of those countries is rather less, that is to say Indonesia and Pakistan are considered low income countries (United Nations [UN] income level 1), whilst Thailand and the Philippines are categorized as middle-income countries (UN level 2). Because of a 2-3 fold higher than IRP price of innovators, it is very difficult for people from low income countries to cope up, people of such countries then end up spending an exhorbitant 77% of the healthcare budget in just buying medicines.

There were three major concerns found in the health care scenario prevailing in UN income level 1 group:

1. Unavailability of the drugs required by people
2. Non affordability to buy medicines because of excessive higher prices quoted as against the IRPs.
3. Unethical medicine promotion

The local government of Indonesia bought the generic medicines at prices 74% greater than the IRP. In Thailand, generic prices were 1.46-fold higher than IRPs, while innovator brands were 3.3 fold higher with regards to public sector. But the scenario with public buying medicines was all the more pathetic. Patients bought branded at 11.60 fold higher prices as compared to IRP and generics at 3.31-fold higher than IRPs. A 15-fold greater than the IRP price in case of innovators, while the lowest-cost generic equivalents were more than 6-fold greater than the IRP for patients buying medicines and a 14- and 15-fold higher than the IRP for branded and generic drugs was the procurement price by the local government of phillipines respectively. Although both Philippines and Thailand both have HTA programmes in place, but it would be more practical if Philippines goes in for other pricing strategies before utilizing pharmacoeconomics. Affordability of medicines can be increased to a large extent by application of appropriate pricing strategies.

Conclusively it can be said that the performance and progress of pharmaceutical sector of a country is equivalent to the socioeconomic and health status. The health status is also considered, because the supply and demand concept applies here.

Following things needs to be taken care of:

- Increasing awareness of Pharmacoeconomics is quintessential.
- Using HTA alone for all medicines as a 'blanket strategy' will not solve the issue of cost containment.
- There are still some countries wherein 77% of the healthcare budget is spent on medicines especially the low income countries.
- Improvement on drug pricing policies.
- Health status and pharmaceutical situation of the country needs to be primarily considered before going ahead to apply pharmacoeconomics strategy.

Pharmaceuticals and other therapeutic interventions have contributed to the significant progress being made in the health care sector of developed and developing countries. Although drugs account for only a diminutive fraction of the expenditures in the hospital budgets, but drug therapy plays a crucial role in the effective treatment of hospitalized patients. This is because a hospitalized patient normally receives around 7-8 drugs on a given day. The fact that the average stay of a patient in hospital have reduced significantly speaks volumes of the efficient drug therapy.

There is a general substantiation supporting the use of pharmaceuticals. But the data in hand pertaining to the actual cost-benefit estimates of drug therapies are very few. Inadequate methodologies to evaluate medical intervention are one of the prime reasons for the lack of such data. Thus, methodologies to not only evaluate the outcomes of drug therapy, but to also put them in perspective of other related healthcare expenditures become essential.

In pharmacoeconomics, results and value of healthcare interventions are expressed by the term outcomes. As mentioned above there is a multidimensional aspect to outcomes, viz: economic, humanistic and clinical. Healthcare administrators and payers are concerned about the economic outcomes of healthcare decisions. Clinical outcomes of the treatment are the main focus with Clinicians. Patients are now becoming increasingly interested in taking their own decisions with regard to their own health care and are inclined towards humanistic outcomes of therapy.

With growing need to strengthen healthcare system and have a successful healthcare management, *i.e.* to satisfy the aims and objectives of patients, physicians, other healthcare providers etc efforts to better the quality of healthcare imparted is also equally important. Thus a holistic healthcare system must necessarily comprise a three dimensional perspective including humanistic and clinical outcomes along with the associated costs or economic consideration. Thus unlike pure economics which is likely to be considered as trade-offs-between goods/services and money, pharmacoeconomics contains both resource utility and humanistic evaluations of drug therapy. Thus the documentation of the degree to which benefits outweigh the costs of healthcare provided is the essence of pharmacoeconomics research or analysis. Hence it is evident that pharmaceutical care alone *i.e.* drugs available for patients to give the necessary therapeutic care is in itself incomplete without pharmacoeconomics per se.

Thus this chapter is basically designed from the point of view to acquaint readers to basic methods used in pharmacoeconomic evaluation. Thus as discussed earlier the various methodologies would be estimation of cost-effectiveness, cost-minimization, cost-benefits, cost-of-illness, cost-utility, cost-consequences, decision analysis, quality of life and other humanistic assessment. This evaluation mechanism thus helps in illustrating the cost impact of innovative treatments and in turn enhancing the acceptance by patients, public and healthcare payers plus administrators.

PHARMACOECONOMIC METHODOLOGIES

Cost-Minimization Analysis

When two or more interventions which have equivalent clinical and humanistic outcomes or consequences are analysed in terms of cost associated with each intervention, such an analysis is cost-minimization analysis. Two generically equivalent drugs in which outcome (*i.e.* therapeutic effect) has been proven to be the same but the purchase and administration costs are visibly different.

Cost minimization analysis can be an exception in case of many clinical applications which are outside true generic substitution.

Cost-Benefit Analysis

In this case all the benefits from an intervention or program are identified and they are then converted into dollars for the year in which they would occur. These dollars which arises due to benefits per year is discounted to its equivalent present value at a chosen interest rate. However it is certainly challenging and rather difficult to measure many benefits, converting them to dollars or both for example: assessing the benefits of improved quality of life experienced by the patient, patient satisfaction with the healthcare system and working conditions of physicians. Hence it is evident that in certain scenarios it is not only difficult to measure the benefits of medical intervention but also it is indeed a task so as to assign a dollar to the benefit identified. Thus as many benefits possible is converted into dollars or monetary units, and the rest of the benefits are labelled as intangible benefits. This kind of analysis is done when there are comparisons done between dissimilar programs, wherein the outcomes are in different units, for example: cancer patient care Vs cardiac rehabilitation program.

Also cost benefit analysis is an answer to more complex problems in that it would permit for assessment of various interventions with dissimilar and multiple outcomes.

Cost-Effectiveness Analysis

As the name suggests, this kind of analysis is done to assist the decision maker in making a preferred choice between available options or altenatives. Health matters where program inputs can be readily estimated in dollars but the programs outputs are more appropriately stated in terms of health improvement created, such matters finds its way into cost effective analysis.

Thus such an analysis is appropriate in cases wherein the outcomes of an intervention are measured in the same terms *i.e.* natural and measurable terms.

Cost-Utility Analysis

This tool enables estimating the consequence of an intervention in terms of quality and quantity of life. It is almost similar to cost-effective analysis with an added facet of patient's point of view. In this case, generally the cost utility analysis is expressed in terms of the intervention cost per quality adjusted life year gained or changes in quality of life measurement for a given intervention cost. Hence cost utility measurements is a gold standard in pharmacoeconomic research, since it takes into acocunt patient preference and quality of life.

Cost of Illness Evaluation

This kind of evaluation is used in case of new therapies. In this case a baseline for comparison is drawn dependent on the impact of the disease and the resources required treating a medical condition prior to discovery of a new intervention. Design and intent of the study remain the two important parameters which are needed in giving a ballpark figure in this type of evaluation.

Cost-Consequence Analysis

In such analysis, the cost and effects are calculated but not aggregated into quality adjusted life years or cost effectiveness ratios. Costs such as direct medical costs, indirect costs, direct nonmedical costs and outcomes like utility impacts and quality of life impacts are evaluated. Healthcare decision makers prefer this analysis since it provides a comprehensive presentation information. But despite the pluses of this analysis, the two drawbacks are listed below:

- Being the discretion of each individual decision makers, it may not be in the society's or patient's best interest.
- Variety of data from clinical trials is also considered, and hence extrapolations and imputations become necessary.

Drug Development and Pharmacoeconomics

Conducting pharmacoeconomic studies during the drug development process can considerably reduce Research and development expenditures. The huge investments going into R & D can be attributed to the many compounds that need to be assessed to bring one drug to the market. It takes around million dollars plus fourteen years of time span spent to bring a novel drug to the market. Thus a pharmacoeconomic evaluation needs to be done in the early stages of drug development process. Hence after an FDA approval is obtained for an investigational new drug application and when a green signal is given to commence the clinical trials (phase I, phase II and phase III) and Phase IV stages of post marketing research, the pharmacoeconomic studies should ideally start as well.

Pharmacoeconomic studies performed during the various stages of life cycle of drug development are mentioned below:

1. ***Phase I trials:*** Toxicity studies are done during phase I of the clinical trials on healthy volunteers. Here the size and frequency of the dose is steadily increased untill the toxic effects surface up. In other words therapeutic dosage exceeds and goes above the maximum safe concentration to show up as toxic effects. At this stage it becomes essential to do a cost of illness evaluation to take a decision on whether to further develop the drug and gather background information for potential pharmacoeconomic evaluations. This kind of an evaluation also enables in the preliminary model development for the clinical benefits expected out of a new intervention in order to have a marketable product.
2. ***Phase II trials:*** In this particular phase, the drug is given to a select few patients having a target disease. To avoid a confounding analysis, to have a better clarity on the drugs activity and to lessen the number of variables, patients without complicating the coexisting medical conditions are preferred here. This enables in a better demonstration of the drugs therapeutic benefit. But this could be a tedious task to prove the efficacy of a new drug even when the patients are carefully selected. Thus to compare the benefit of the new drug with that of the standard treatments available in market becomes really essential to provide an indisputable confirmation of the drugs therapeutic benefit. Cost of illness studies can either begin or continue in this phase.
3. ***Phase III trials:*** Phase III trials help in identifying rare reactions shown by patients which is caused by the new drug. This is because the new drug in the established dosage form, dose and frequency is given to a larger sample size. Discussion, plannning and implementation of pharmacoeconomic studies during this level of research is very important.

4. ***Phase IV trials:*** In all the previous trials, *i.e.* Phase I–Phase III, the evaluation of costs and benefits is performed in strictly controlled situation and nor real world environment. This is because such an evaluation only delas with the drug's efficacy which is "can it work"? and not effectiveness *i.e.* "does it work"?. Cost effectiveness parameter can be confirmed only when the product enters the market. Thus PE studies done during the post marketing or phase IV trials, throws light on the effectivness part of the drug therapy. Both retrospective *i.e.* evaluations done based on information from previous clinical trials and prospective studies can be done during this phase of the clinical trial studies.

The threefold link between pharmacoeconomic evaluation and clinical trials are as mentioned below:

- Pharmacoeconomic evaluation may be a secondary purpose to a clinical trial
- PE evaluation may be done retrospectively utilising clincial data from the previous studies.
- PE may also be the chief purpose for which a clinical trial is conducted.

Just as it is unfeasible to develop an algorithm for the treatment of a disease that is suitable for all patients suffering from a particular disease, it is equally impossible to develop one for making pharmacoeconomic decision.

References

1. Waller, P.C. (1998). Pharmacovigilance towards the next millennium. *Br. J. Clin. Pharmacol.,* 45(5): 417.
2. Meyboom, R.H., Egberts, A.C., Edwards, I.R., Hekster, Y.A., de Koning, F.H. and Gribnau, F.W. (1997). Principles of signal detection in pharmacovigilance. *Drug Safety: An International Journal of Medical Toxicology and Drug Experience*. 16(6): 355–65.
3. Meyboom, R.H., Hekster, Y.A., Egberts, A.C., Gribnau, F.W. and Edwards, I.R. (1997). Causal or Casual? The role of causality assessment in Pharmacovigilance. *Drug Safety: An International Journal of Medical Toxicology and Drug Experience*. 17(6): 374–89.
4. Simon, L.S. (2002). Pharmacovigilance: Towards a better understanding of the benefit to risk ratio. *Ann, Rheum Dis.,* 61(2): 88–89.
5. http://www.mhra.gov.uk/Howweregulate/Medicines/Licensingofmedicines/Informationforlicenceapplicants/PeriodicSafetyUpdateReports/index.htm; accessed 15th March 2012.
6. Benichou, C. (1994). Adverse drug reactions: A Practical guide to diagnosis and management: Imputability of unexpected or toxic drug reactions. New York: JohnWiley& Sons.
7. Edwards, I.R. (2001). Drug benefits and risks, International text book of Clinical Pharmacology: Adverse Drug Reactions. Wiley & Sons.
8. Wilson, A.M., Thabane, L. and Holbrook, A. (2004). Application of data mining techniques in Pharmacovigilance. *Br. J. Clin. Pharmacol.*, 57(2):127–134.
9. (2004). WHO. Policy Perspectives on Medicines. Pharmacovigilance: Ensuring the safe use of medicines Geneva, World Health Organization.
10. (2000). WHO. Safety monitoring of medicnes. Guidelines for setting up and running a pharmacovigilance centre. Geneva, World Health Organization.
11. (1998). WHO. Effective communications in pharmacovigilance: The Erice Report. Uppsala. World Health Organization Collaborating Centre for International Drug Monitoring.
12. (2002). WHO. Expecting the worst. Anticipating, preventing and managing medicinal product crises. Uppsala, World Health Organization Collaborating Centre for International Drug Monitoring.
13. Van Boxtel, C.J., Santoso, B. and Edwards, I.R. (*eds*) (2001). International textbook of clinical pharmacology: Drug benefits and risks. Chichester: John Wiley & Sons.

14. Pirmohamed, M.K., Atuah, K.N., Dodoo, A.N.O. and Winstanley, P. (2007). Pharmacovigilance in developing countries. *Br. Med. J.,* 335: 462.
15. Lazarou, J., Pomeranz, B. and Corey, P. (1998). Incidence of adverse raections in hospitalized patients: A meta–analyis of prospective studies. *Journal of the American Medical Association*. 279(15): 1200–05.
16. Edwards, I.R. and Aronson, J.K. (2000). Adverse drug reactions: Definitions, diagnosis, and management. *Lancet*. 356: 1255–9.
17. Fountoulakis, M., Berndt, P. and Boelsterli, U.A. (2000). Two–dimensional database of mouse liver proteins: Changes in hepatic protein levels following treatment with acetaminophen or its nontoxic regioisomer 3–acetamidophenol. *Electrophoresis.,* 21: 2148–61.
18. Dodd, C.C., Naisbitt, D.J., Vilar, F.J. *et al.* (2003). Abacavir hypersensitivity in human immunodeficiency virus positive patients: Demonstration of the presence of drug–specific lymphocyte proliferation *in vitro*. *Br. J. Clin. Pharmacol.,* 55: 421.
19. Mamdani, M., Juurlink, D.N., Lee, D.S. *et al.* (2004). Cyclooxygenase– 2 inhibitors versus non–selective non steroidal anti–inflammatory drugs and congestive heart failure outcomes in elderly patients: A population based cohort study. *Lancet*. 363: 1751–6.
20. Cleland, J.G.F., Dargie, J.H., McAlpine, H. *et al.* (1985). Severe hypotension after first dose of enalapril in the elderly. *Br. Med. J.,* 291: 1309–12.
21. Alfirevic, A., Mills, T., Harrington, P. *et al.* (2006). Serious carbamazepine–induced hypersensitivity reactions associated with the HSP70 gene cluster. *Pharmacogenet Genomics*. 16: 287–96.
22. Descamps, V., Valance, A., Edlinger, C. *et al.* (2001). Association of human herpesvirus 6 infection with drug reaction with eosinophilia and systemic symptoms. *Arch Dermatol.,* 137: 301–4.
23. Anderson, C.C. and Matzinger, P. (2000). Danger: The view from the bottom of the cliff. *Semin Immunol.,* 12: 231–8.
24. Bates, D.W., Spell, N., Cullen, D.J. *et al.* (1997). The costs of adverse drug events in hospitalized patients. *JAMA*. 277: 307–11.
25. Mirochnitchenko, O., Weisbrot–Lefkowitz, M., Reuhl, K. *et al.* (1999). Acetaminophen toxicity. Opposite effects of two forms of glutathione peroxidase. *J. Biol. Chem.,* 274: 10349–55.
26. Fries, S., Grosser, T., Price, T.S. *et al.* (2006). Marked interindividual variability in the response to selective inhibitors of cyclooxygenase–2. *Gastroenterology*. 130: 55–64.
27. Henderson, C.J., Wolf, C.R., Kitteringham, N. *et al.* (2000). Increased resistance to acetaminophen hepatotoxicity in mice lacking glutathione S–transferase Pi. *Proc. Natl. Acad Sci. U S A*. 97: 12741–5.
28. Hetherington, S., Hughes, A.R., Mosteller, M. *et al.* (2002). Genetic variations in HLA–B region and hypersensitivity reactions to abacavir. *Lancet.* 359: 1121–2.
29. Petty, G.W., Brown, R.D., Whisnant, J.P. *et al.* (1999). Frequency of major complications of aspirin, warfarin, and intravenous heparin for secondary stroke prevention – A population–based study. *Ann Intern Med.,* 130: 14–22.

30. Brown, E.G. (2004). Using MedDRA: Implications for risk management. *Drug Safety*. 27(8): 591–602.
31. Orme, M., Harry, J., Routledge, P. and Hobson, S. (1989). Healthy volunteer studies in Great Britain: The results of a survey into 12 months activity in this field. *Br. J. Clin. Pharmacol.,* 27: 125–33.
32. Purkins, L., Love, E.R., Eve, M.D., Wooldridge, C.L., Cowan, C., Smart, T.S., Johnson, P.J. and Rapeport, W.G. (2004). The influence of diet upon liver function tests and serum lipids in healthy male volunteers resident in a Phase I unit. *Br. J. Clin. Pharmacol.,* 57(2): 199–208.
33. Lin, Y.L., Chern, H.D. and Chu, M.L. (2003). Hepatotoxicity in the review of clinical safety data. *Drug Inf. J.,* 37: 155–8.
34. Ott, E., Nussmeier, N.A., Duke, P.C. *et al.* (2003). Multicenter study of perioperative ischemia research group and the ischemia research and education foundation investigators. Efficacy and safety of the cyclooxygenase 2 inhibitors parecoxib and valdecoxib in patients undergoing coronary bypass surgery. *Journal of Thoracic and Cardiovascular Surgery*. 125: 1481–92.
35. Naisbitt, D.J., Britschgi, M., Wong, G. *et al.* (2003). Hypersensitivity reactions to carbamazepine: Characterization of the specificity, phenotype and cytokine profile of drugspecific T cell clones. *Mol. Pharmacol.,* 63: 732–41.
36. Malucchi, S., Capobianco, M., Gilli, F., Marnetto, F., Caldano, M., Sala, A. and Bertolotto, A. (2005). Fate of multiple sclerosis patients positive for neutralising antibodies towards interferon beta shifted to alternative treatments. *Neurol. Sci.,* 4: S213–S214,
37. Pirmohamed, M., Alfirevic, A., Vilar, J. *et al.* (2000). Association analysis of drug metabolizing enzyme gene polymorphisms in HIV–positive patients with co–trimoxazole hypersensitivity. *Pharmacogenetics*. 10: 705–13.
38. Hamdy, R.C., Murnane, B. and Perera, N. (1982). Pharmacokinetics of benoxaprofen in elderly subjects. *Eur. J. Rheumatol. Infamm.,* 5: 69–76.
39. Pirmohamed, M. (2006). Genetic factors in the predisposition to drug–induced hypersensitivity reactions. *AAPSJ*. 8(1): E20–6.
40. Groen, H., Horan, M.A. and Roberts, N.A. (1993). The relationship between phenazone (antipyrine) metabolite formation and theophylline metabolism in healthy and frail elderly women. *Clin Pharmacokinet.,* 25: 136–44.
41. Pirmohamed, M., Kitteringham, N.R., Guenthner, T.M. *et al.* (1992). An investigation of the formation of cytotoxic, protein–reactive and stable metabolites from carbamazepine *in vitro*. *Biochem. Pharmacol.*, 43: 1675–82.
42. Pessayre, D. and Larrey, D. (1988). Acute and chronic drug–induced hepatitis. *Baillieres Clin Gastroenterol.,* 2: 385–422.
43. Merten, G.J., Burgess, W.P., Gray, L.V. *et al.* (2004). Prevention of contrast–induced nephropathy with sodium bicarbonate: A randomized controlled trial. *JAMA*. 291(19): 2328–34.
44. Nash, K., Hafeez, A. and Hou, S. (2002). Hospital–acquired renal insufficiency. *Am. J. Kidney Dis.,* 39(5): 930–6.
45. Vlahakos, D.V., Manginas, A., Chilidou, D. *et al.* (2002). Itraconazole–induced rabdomyolysis and acute renal failure in a heart transplant recipient treated with simvastatin and cyclosporine. *Transplantation*, 73: 1962–4.

46. (2001). The International SNP Map Working Group. A map of human genome sequence variation containing 1.42 million single nucleotide polymorphisms. *Nature*. 409: 928–33.
47. Ray, S.D., Sorge, C.L., Raucy, J.L. and Corcoran, G.B. (1990). Early loss of large genomic DNA *in vivo* with accumulation of Ca^{2+} in the nucleus during acetaminophen–induced liver injury. *Toxicol. Appl. Pharmacol.,* 106: 346–51.
48. Tsokos–Kuhn, J.O. (1989). Evidence *in vivo* for elevation of intracellular free Ca^{2+} in the liver after diquat, acetaminophen, and CCl4. *Biochem. Pharmacol.,* 38: 3061–5.
49. Sloane, P.D., Zimmerman, S., Brown, L.C. *et al.* (2002). Inappropriate medication prescribing in residential care/assisted living facilities. *J. Am. Geriatr Soc.,* 50: 1001–11.
50. Sharief, M.K. and Hentges, R. (1991). Association between tumor necrosis factor–alpha and disease progression in patients with multiple sclerosis. *N. Engl. J. Med.,* 325: 467–72.
51. Honig, P.K., Wortham, D.C., Zamani, K. *et al.* (1993). Terfenadine–keto–conazole interaction: Pharmacokinetic and electrocardiographic consequences. *J. Am. Med. Assoc.,* 269: 513–18.
52. Wadelius, M., Chen, L.Y., Downes, K. *et al.* (2005). Common VKORC1 and GGCX polymorphisms associated with warfarin dose. *Pharmacogenomics J.*, 5: 262–70.
53. Zhang, H., Cook, J., Nickel. J. *et al.* (2000). Reduction of liver Fas expression by an antisense oligonucleotide protects mice from fulminant hepatitis. *Nat. Biotechnol.,* 18: 862–7.
54. Moinova, H.R. and Mulcahy, R.T. (1998). An electrophile responsive element (EpRE) regulates betanaphthoflavone induction of the human gammaglutamylcysteine synthetase regulatory subunit gene. Constitutive expression is mediated by an adjacent AP–1 site. *J. Biol. Chem.,* 273: 14683–9.
55. Onder, G., Pedone, C., Landi, F. *et al.* (2002). Adverse drug reactions as cause of hospital admissions: Results from the Italian Group of Pharmacoepidemiology in the Elderly (GIFA). *J. Am. Geriatr Soc.,* 50: 1962–8.
56. Martin, A.M., Nolan, D., Gaudieri, S. *et al.* (2004). Predisposition to abacavir hypersensitivity conferred by HLAB*5701 and a haplotypic Hsp70–Hom variant. *Proc. Natl. Acad. Sci. USA,* 101: 4180–5.
57. Robertson, J.S. (2006). Changes in biological source material. *Biologicals*. 34: 61–63.
58. Mertes, P.M. and Laxenaire, M.C. (2002). Allergic reactions occurring during anaesthesia. *European Journal of Anaesthesiology*. 19: 240–62.
59. Perrier, N.D., Baerga–Varela, Y. and Murray, M.J. (2000). Death related to propofol use in an adult patient. *Crit. Care Med.,* 28: 3071–4.
60. Miller, J., Chan, B.K.S. and Nelson, H. (2002). Postmenopausal estrogen replacement and risk for venous thromboembolism: A systematic review and meta–analysis for the US Preventive Services Task Force. *Ann. Intern. Med.,* 136: 680–90.

61. Pouyanne, P., Haramburu, F. and Imbs, J.L. (2000). Begaud B for the French Pharmacovigilance centres. Admissions to hospital caused by adverse drug reactions: Cross sectional incidence study. *BMJ*. 320: 1036.
62. Ingelman–Sundberg, M., Oscarson, M. and McLellan, R.A. (1999). Polymorphic human cytochrome P450 enzymes: An opportunity for individualized drug treatment. *Trends Pharmacol Sci.,* 20: 342–9.
63. Grandison, M.K. and Boudinot, F.D. (2000). Age–related changes in protein binding of drugs: Implications for therapy. *Clin. Pharmacokinet,* 38(3): 271–90.
64. Hetherington, S, McGuirk, S., Powell, G. *et al.* (2001). Hypersensitivity reactions during therapy with the nucleoside reverse transcriptase inhibitor abacavir. *Clin. Ther.,* 23: 1603–14.
65. Hanlon, J.T., Lindblad, C.I., Hajjir, E. and McCarthy, T.C. (2003). Update on drug–related problems in the elderly. *Am. J. Geriatr Pharmacother,* 1: 38–43.
66. Mallal, S., Nolan, D., Witt, C. *et al.* (2002). Association between presence of HLA– B*5701, HLA–DR7 and HLADQ3 and hypersensitivity to HIV–1 reverse transcriptase inhibitor abacavir. *Lancet*, 359: 727–32.
67. Reicin, A., Shapiro, D., Sperling, R.S. *et al.* (2002). Comparison of cardiovascular thrombotic events in patients with osteoarthritis treated with Rofecoxib vs nonselective non–steroidal antiinflammatory drugs (ibuprofen, diclofenac and nabumetone). *American Journal of Cardiology*. 89: 204–9.
68. Mauri–Hellweg, D., Bettens, F., Mauri, D. *et al.* (1995). Activation of drug–specific CD4_+_ and CD8_+_ T–cells in individuals allergic to sulfonamides, phenytoin, and carbamazepine. *J. Immunol.,* 155: 462–72.
69. Hrachovec, J.B. and Mora, M. (2001). Reporting of 6–month vs 12–month data in a clinical trial and celecoxib. *JAMA*. 286: 2398–400.
70. Raucy, J.L., Lasker, J.M., Lieber, C.S. and Black, M. (1989). Acetaminophen activation by human liver cytochromes P–450IIE1 and P–450IA2. *Arch. Biochem. Biophys.,* 271: 270–83.
71. Hale, W., Stewart, R.B. and Marks, R.G. (1985). Antianxiety drugs and central nervous system symptoms in an ambulatory elderly population. *Drug Intell Clin. Pharm.,* 19: 37–40.
72. Chu, L.W. and Pei, C.K. (1999). Risk factors for early emergency hospital readmission in elderly medical patients. *Gerontology*. 45: 220–6.
73. Park, B.K., Coleman, J.W. and Kitteringham, N.R. (1987). Drug disposition and drug hypersensitivity. *Biochem. Pharmacol.,* 36: 581–90.
74. Moinova, H.R. and Mulcahy, R.T. (1998). An electrophile responsive element (EpRE) regulates betanaphthoflavone induction of the human gammaglutamylcysteine synthetase regulatory subunit gene. Constitutive expression is mediated by an adjacent AP–1 site. *J. Biol. Chem.,* 273: 14683–9.
75. Hughes, D.A., Vilar, F.J., Ward, C.C. *et al.* (2004). Costeffectiveness analysis of HLA B*5701 genotyping in preventing abacavir hypersensitivity. *Pharmacogenetics*. 14: 335–42.
76. Schellekens, H. (2004). Biosimilar therapeutic agents: Issues with bioequivalence and immunogenicity. *Eur. J. Clin. Invest.,* 34: 797–799.

77. Graham, D.J., Campen, D., Hui, R. *et al.* (2005). Risk of acute myocardial infarction and sudden cardiac death in patients treated with cyclo–oxygenase 2 selective and nonselective non–steroidal anti–inflammatory drugs: Nested case–control study. *Lancet*. 365: 475–81.
78. Kitteringham, N.R., Powell, H., Clement, Y.N. *et al.* (2000). Hepatocellular response to chemical stress in CD–1 mice: Induction of early genes and gamma–glutamylcysteine synthetase. *Hepatology*. 32: 321–33.
79. Carr, A. and Cooper, D.A. (1995). Pathogenesis and management of HIV–associated drug hypersensitivity. *AIDS Clin. Rev.,* 96: 65–97.
80. Haining, R.L., Hunter, A.P., Veronese, M.E. *et al.* (1996). Allelic variants of human cytochrome P450 2C9: Baculovirusmediated expression, purification, structural characterization, substrate stereoselectivity, and prochiral selectivity of the wild–type and I359L mutant forms. *Arch. Biochem. Biophys.,* 333: 447–58.
81. Ray, W.A., Stein, C.M., Daugherty, J.R. *et al.* (2002). COX–2 selective non-steroidal anti–inflammatory drugs and risk of serious coronary heart disease. *Lancet,* 360: 1071–3.
82. Clark, D.W. (2004). Harrison–Woolrych ML. Sibutramine may be associated with memory impairment. *BMJ*, 329: 1316.
83. Faucheron, J.L. (1999). Toxicity of non–steroidal anti–inflammatory drugs in the large bowel. *Eur. J. Gastroenterol. Hepatol,* 11: 389–92.
84. (1993). International Conference on Harmonisation (ICH) Expert Working Group E7. Studies in support of special populations. *Geriatrics,* 111: 3388–93.
85. Lee, S.S.T., Buters, J.T.M., Pineau, T. *et al.* (1996). Role of cyp2e1 in the hepatotoxicity of acetaminophen. *J. Biol. Chem.,* 271: 12063–7.
86. Mirochnitchenko, O., Weisbrot–Lefkowitz, M., Reuhl, K. *et al.* (1999). Acetaminophen toxicity. Opposite effects of two forms of glutathione peroxidase. *J. Biol. Chem.,* 274: 10349–55.
87. Park, B.K., Kitteringham, N.R., Maggs, J.L. *et al.* (2005). The role of metabolic activation in drug–induced hepatotoxicity. *Annu. Rev. Pharmacol. Toxicol,* 45: 177–202.
88. Michalets, E.L. and Williams, C.R. (2000). Drug interactions with cisapride: Clinical implications. *Clin. Pharmacokinet,* 39: 49–75.
89. Brynne, N., Forslund, C., Hallen, B. *et al.* (1999). Ketoconazole inhibits the metabolism of tolterodine in subjects with deficient CYP2D6 activity. *Br. J. Clin. Pharmacol.,* 48: 564–72.
90. Gurwitz, J.H. (2004). Polypharmacy – a new paradigm for quality drug therapy in the elderly? *Arch. Intern. Med.,* 164: 1957–9.
91. Clarke, A., Deeks, J.J., Shakir, S.A.W. (2006). An assessment of the publicly disseminated evidence of safety used in decisions to withdraw medicinal products from the UK and US markets. *Drug Saf.,* 29: 175–81.
92. Bigger, J.T. (1982). The quinidine–digoxin interaction. *Mod. Concepts Cardiovasc Dis..* 51: 73–8.
93. Castleden, C.M. and Pickles, H. (1988). Suspected adverse drug reactions in elderly patients reported to the CSM. *Br. J. Clin. Pharmacol.,* 26: 347–53.

94. Fossa, A.A., Depasquale, M.J., Raunig, D.L. *et al.* (2002). The relationship of clinical QT prolongation to outcome in the conscious dog using a beat–to–beat QT–RR interval assessment. *J. Pharmacol. Exp. Ther.,* 202: 828–33.
95. Aptula, A.O. and Cronin, M.T. (2004). Prediction of hERG K+ blocking potency: Application of structural knowledge. *SAR QSAR Environ. Res.,* 15: 399–411.
96. FitzGerald, G.A. (2004). Coxibs and cardiovascular disease. New England *Journal of Medicine.* 351: 1709–11.
97. Joshi, A., Dimino, T., Vohra, Y. *et al.* (2004). Preclinical strategies to assess QT liability and torsadogenic potential of new drugs: The role of experimental models. *J. Electrocardiol.,* 37(Suppl): 7–14.
98. Venot, A. (1999). Electronic prescribing for the elderly: Will it improve medication usage? *Drug Aging.,* 15: 77–80.
99. Natsukawa, T., Matsuzaki, T., Hayashi, S. *et al.* (1998). Comparison of the effects of NS–21 and terodiline on the QTc interval in dogs. *Gen. Pharmacol.,* 30: 137–42.
100. Gurwitz, J.H., Goldberg, R.J., Holden, A. *et al.* (1998). Agerelated risks of long–term oral anti–coagulant therapy. *Arch. Intern. Med.,* 148: 1733–6.
101. Haverkamp, W., Breithardt, G., Camm, A.J. *et al.* (2000). The potential for QT prolongation and proarrhythmia by nonantiarrhythmic drugs: Clinical and regulatory implications. Report on a Policy Conference of the European Society of Cardiology. *Eur Heart J.,* 21: 1216–31.
102. Sanguinetti, M.C. and Mitcheson, J.S. (2005). Predicting drug ERG channel interactions that cause acquired long QT syndrome. *Trends Pharmacol. Sci.,* 26: 119–24.
103. Israel, B.C., Blouin, R.A., McIntyre, W. and Shedlofsky, S.T. (1993). Effects of interferon–alphamonotherapy on hepatic drug metabolism in cancer patients. *Br. J. Clin. Pharmacol.,* 36: 229–35.
104. Schepkens, H., Vanholder, R., Billiouw, J.M. and Lameire, N. (2001). Life–threatening hyperkalemia during combined therapy with angiotensin–converting enzyme inhibitors and spironolactone: An analysis of 25 cases. *Am. J. Med.,* 110(6): 438–41.
105. Verhulst, A., D'Haese, P.C. and De Broe, M.E. (2004). Inhibitors of HMG–CoA reductase reduce receptor–mediated endocytosis in human kidney proximal tubular cells. *J. Am. Soc. Nephrol.,* 15(9): 2249–57.
106. Moghal, N.E., Brocklebank, J.T., Meadow, S.R. (1998). A review of acute renal failure in children: Incidence, etiology and outcome. *Clin. Nephrol,* 49(2): 91–5.
107. Riker, R.R. and Fraser, G.L. (2005). Adverse events associated with prolonged use of sedatives, analgesics, and other drugs that provide patient comfort in the intensive care unit. *Pharmacotherapy.* 25: 8S–18S.
108. Geelen, P., Drolet, B., Rail, J. *et al.* (2000). Sildenafil (Viagra) prolongs cardiac repolarization by blocking the rapid component of the delayed rectifier potassium current. *Circulation.* 102: 275–7.
109. Yang, P., Kanki, H., Drolet, B. *et al.* (2002). Allelic variants in long–QT disease genes in patients with drug associated torsades de pointes. *Circulation,* 105: 1943–8.

110. Tomaselli, G.F. and Zipes, D.P. (2004). What causes sudden death in heart failure? *Circ. Res.,* 95: 754–63.
111. Belsey, M.J., Harris, L.M., Das, R.R. and Chertkow, J. (2006). Biosimilars: Initial excitement gives way to reality. *Nat. Rev. Drug Discov.,* 5:535–536.
112. Sloane, P.D., Gruber–Baldini, A.L., Zimmerman, S. *et al.* (2004). Medication undertreatment in assisted living settings. *Arch. Intern. Med.,* 164: 2031–7.
113. Gribbin, B., Pickering, T.G., Sleight, P. and Peto, R. (1971). Effect of age and high blood pressure on baroreceptor sensitivity in man. *Circ Res.,* 29: 424–31.
114. Recanatini, M., Poluzzi, E., Masetti, M. *et al.* (2005). QT prolongation through hERG K+ channel blockade: Current knowledge and strategies for the early prediction during drug development. *Med. Res. Rev.,* 25: 133–66.
115. Postlind, H., Danielson, A., Lindgren, A. and Andersson, S.H.G. (1998). Tolterodine, a new muscarinic receptor antagonist, is metabolized by cytochromes P450 2D6 and 3A in human liver microsomes. *Drug Metab Dispos.*, 26: 289–93.
116. Noren, B., Stromberg, S., Ericsson, O. and Lindeke, B. (1989). Biotransformation of terodiline V. Stereoselectivity in hydroxylation by human liver microsomes. *Chem. Biol. Interactions,* 71: 325–37.
117. Layton, D., Key, C. and Shakir, S.A. (2003). Prolongation of the QT interval and cardiac arrhythmias associated with cisapride: Limitations of the pharmacoepidemiological studies conducted and proposals for the future. *Pharmacoepidemiol Drug Saf.*, 12: 31–40.
118. Hartigan–Go, K., Bateman, N.D. and Daly, A.K. (1996). Thomas SHL. Stereoselective cardiotoxic effects of terodiline. *Clin. Pharmacol. Ther.,* 60: 89–98.
119. Fischer–Rasmussen, W. (1984). Evaluation of long–term safety and clinical benefit of terodiline in women with urgency/urge incontinence. A multicentre study. *Scand. J. Urol. Nephrol. Suppl.,* 87: 35–47.
120. Matchaba, P., Gitton, X., Krammer, G. *et al.* (2005). Cardiovascular safety of lumiracoxib: A meta–analysis of all randomized controlled trials e"1 week and up to 1 year in duration of patients with osteoarthritis and rheumatoid arthritis. *Clinical Therapeutics,* 27: 1196–214.
121. Andersson, K.E., Ekstrom, B. and Mattiasson, A. (1988). Actions of terodiline, its isomers and main metabolite on isolated detrusor muscle from rabbit and man. *Pharmacol. Toxicol.,* 63: 390–5.
122. Venulet, J. (1986). Incomplete information as a limiting factor in causality assessment of adverse drug reactions and its practical consequences. *Drug Information Journal,* 20: 423–31.
123. Klepper, M.J. (2004). The periodic safety update report as a pharmacovigilance tool. *Drug Safety,* 27(8): 569–78.
124. Brynne, N., Forslund, C., Hallen, B. *et al.* (1999). Ketoconazole inhibits the metabolism of tolterodine in subjects with deficient CYP2D6 activity. *Br. J. Clin. Pharmacol.,* 1999; 48: 564–72.
125. Aronov, A.M. (2005). Predictive in silico modeling for hERG channel blockers. *Drug Discov. Today,* 10: 149–55.

126. Geelen, P., Drolet, B., Rail, J. *et al.* (2000). Sildenafil (Viagra) prolongs cardiac repolarization by blocking the rapid component of the delayed rectifier potassium current. *Circulation*. 102: 275–7.
127. Morganroth, J., Ilson, B.E., Shaddinger, B.C. *et al.* (2004). Evaluation of vardenafil and sildenafil on cardiac repolarization. *Am. J. Cardiol.,* 93: 1378–83.
128. (2003). Food and Drug Administration. 21 CFR Parts 310, 312, *et al.* Safety Reporting Requirements for Human Drug and Biological Products; Proposed Rule. Federal Register, March 14, 2003.
129. Brown, E.G., Wood, K.L. and Wood, S.M. (1999). The medical dictionary for regulatory activities (MedDRA) leading article. *Drug Saf.*, 20(2): 109–17.
130. McGettigan, P., Han, P. and Henry, D. (2006). Cyclooxygenase–2 inhibitors and coronary occlusion: Exploring dose–response relationships. *British Journal of Clinical Pharmacology*. 62: 358–65.
131. Mannesse, C.K., Derkx, F.H., De Ridder, M.A. *et al.* (2000). Contribution of adverse drug reactions to hospital admission of older patients. *Age Ageing.*, 29: 35–9.
132. Kubler, J., Vonk, R., Beimel, S. *et al.* (2005). Adverse event analysis and MedDRA: Business as usual or challenge? *Drug Information Journal*. 39: 63–72.
133. Brown, E.G. (2004). Using MedDRA: Implications for risk management. *Drug Saf.,* 27(8): 591–602.
134. Li, J., Yang, C., Xia, Y., Bertino, A., Glaspy, J., Roberts, M. and Kuter, D.J. (2001). Thrombocytopenia caused by the development of antibodies to thrombopoietin. *Blood,* 98: 3241–3248.
135. Bousquet, C., Lagier, G., Lillo–Le Louet, A. *et al.* (2005). Appraisal of the MedDRA conceptual structure for describing and grouping adverse drug reactions. *Drug Saf.,* 28(1): 19–34.
136. Inui, K.I., Masuda, S. and Saito, H. (2000). Cellular and molecular aspects of drug transport in the kidney. *Kidney Int.,* 58: 944–58.
137. (2005). Proposal for revision of a guideline on summary of product characteristics committee for medicinal products for Human Use. EMEA/ CHMP/64302/2005. Accessed via http://pharmacos.eudra.org.
138. (2005). MedDRA and product labeling: 'Best Practices' Recommendations. MedDRA Maintenance and Support Services Organization,. Accessed via http:/ /www.meddramsso.com.
139. ICH Harmonised Tripartite Guideline: The Common Technical Document for the Registration of Pharmaceuticals for Human Use: Efficacy – M4E, 2005, accessed via http://www.ich.org.
140. Berry, S.J., Coffey, D.S., Walsh, P.C. and Ewing, LL. (1984). The development of human benign prostatic hyperplasia with age. *J. Urol.,* 132: 474–9.
141. Wilton, L.V., Heeley, E., Pickering, R.M. *et al.* (2001). Comparative study of mortality rates and cardiac arrhythmias in post–marketing surveillance studies of sertindole and two other atypical antipsychotic drugs, risperidone and olangipine. *J. Psychopharmacol.,* 15(2): 120–6.
142. Layton, D., Clark, D., Pearce, G. *et al.* (2001). Is there an association between Selective Serotonin Reuptake Inhibitors (SSRI) and the risk of abnormal

bleeding? Results from a cohort study based on prescription event monitoring in England. *Eur. J. Clin. Pharmacol.,* 57(2): 167–76.

143. MacKay, F. (1998). Postmarketing studies: The value of the work of the Drug Safety Research Unit. *Drug Saf.*, 19: 343–53.
144. Coulter, D.M. (2001). Privacy issues and the monitoring of sumatriptan in the New Zealand Intensive Medicines Monitoring Programme. *Pharmacoepidemiol Drug Saf.,* 10: 663–7.
145. Kubler, J., Vonk, R., Beimel, S. *et al.* (2005). Adverse event analysis and MedDRA: Business as usual or challenge? *Drug Information Journal,* 39: 63–72.
146. Kaufman, D.W., Kelly, J.P, Rosenberg, L. *et al.* (2002). Recent patterns of medication use in the ambulatory adult population of the United States. *JAMA,* 287: 337–44.
147. Williams, A. and Denham, M.J. (1998). The ethics of biomedical research in the elderly. *In*: George, C.F., Woodhouse, K.W., Denham, M.J., MacLennan, W.J. *Eds*, Drug Therapy in Old Age. Chichester: Wiley.
148. Juurlink, D.N., Mamdani, M.M., Lee, D.S. *et al.* (2004). Rates of hyperkalemia after publication of the randomized aldactone evaluation study. *N. Engl. J. Med.,* 351(6): 543–51.
149. Levey, A.S., Bosch, J.P., Lewis, J.B. *et al.* (1999). A more accurate method to estimate glomerular filtration rate from serum creatinine: A new prediction equation. Modification of Diet in Renal Disease Study Group. *Ann. Intern. Med.,* 130(6): 461–70.
150. Vercauteren, S.R., Bosmans, J.L., Elseviers, M.M. *et al.* (1998). A meta–analysis and morphological review of cyclosporineinduced nephrotoxicity in auto–immune disease. *Kidney Int.*, 54(2): 536–45.
151. Anon. (1998). HIV adverse drug reactions reporting scheme. *Current Problems in Pharmacovigilance*. 24: 3.
152. Fitz Gerald, G.A. (2003). COX–2 and beyond: Approaches to prostaglandin inhibition in human disease. *Nature Review of Drug Discovery*. 2: 879–90.
153. Fromm, M.F., Kim, R.B., Stein, C.M. *et al.* (1999). Inhibition of P–glycoprotein–mediated drug transport: A unifying mechanism to explain the interaction between digoxin and quinidine. *Circulation,* 99: 552–7.
154. Hall, M., McCormack, P., Arthurs, N. *et al.* (1995). The spontaneous reporting of adverse drug reactions by nurses. *Br. J. Clin. Pharmacol.,* 40: 173–5.
155. Houghton, J., Woods, F., Davis, S. *et al.* (1999). Community pharmacist reporting of suspected ADRs: (2) Attitudes of community pharmacists and general practitioners in Wales. *Pharmacol. J.*, 263: 788–91.
156. Moore, N., Paux, G., Begaud, B. *et al.* (1985). Adverse drug reaction monitoring: Doing it the French way. *Lancet,* 9: 1056–8.
157. Eland, I.A., Belton, K.J., van Grootheest, A.C. *et al.* (1999). Attitudinal survey of voluntary reporting of adverse reactions. *Br. J. Clin. Pharmacol.,* 48: 623–7.
158. Gislason, G.H., Jacobsen, S., Rasmussen, J.N. *et al.* (2006). Risk of death or reinfarction associated with the use of selective cyclooxygenase–2 inhibitors and nonselective nonsteroidal antiinflammatory drugs after acute myocardial infarction. *Circulation*. 113: 2906–13.

159. Hippisley–Cox, J. and Coupland, C. (2005). Risk of myocardial infarction in patients taking cyclooxygenase inhibitors or conventional non–steroidal anti-inflammatory drugs: Population based nested case–control analysis. *BMJ,* 330: 1366–72.
160. Hajjar, E.R., Hanlon, J.T., Artz, M.B. *et al.* (2003). Adverse drug reaction risk factors in older outpatients. *Am. J. Geriatr Pharmacother,* 1: 82–9.
161. Mets, T.F. (1995). Drug–induced orthostatic hypotension in older patients. *Drugs Ageing,* 6: 219–28.
162. Chan, T.Y.K. and Critchley, J.A.J.H. (1994). Reporting of adverse drug reactions in relation to general medical admissions to a teaching hospital in Hong Kong. *Pharmacoepidemiology and Drug Saf.*, 3:85–9.
163. Morrison–Griffiths, S., Walley, T.J., Park, B.K. *et al.* (2003). Reporting of adverse drug reaction by nurses. *Lancet.* 361: 1347–8.
164. Waller, P.C. and Evans, S.J. (2003). A model for the future conduct of pharmacovigilance. *Pharmacoepidemiol Drug Saf.*, 12(1): 17–29.
165. Sweis, D. and Wong, I.C.K. (2000). A survey on factors that could affect adverse drug reaction reporting according to hospital pharmacists in Great Britain. *Drug Saf.,* 23: 165–72.
166. Britt, R.P., James, A.H., Raskino, C.L. and Thompson, S.G. (1992). Factors affecting the precision of warfarin treatment. *J. Clin. Pathol.,* 45: 1003–6.
167. Leeder, J.S. (1996). Developmental aspects of drug metabolism in children. *Drug Inf. J.,* 30: 1135–43.
168. Tsintis, P. and LaMache, E. (2004). CIOMS and ICH initiatives in pharmacovigilance and risk management: Overview and implications. *Drug Safety*. 27: 509–17.
169. Jefferys, D.B., Leakey, D., Lewis, J. *et al.* (1998). New active substances authorized in the United Kingdom between 1972 and 1994. *British Journal of Clinical Pharmacology*. 45: 151–6.
170. Farkouh, M.E., Kirshner, H., Harrington, R.A. *et al.* (2004). On behalf of the TARGET Study Group. Comparison of lumiracoxib with naproxen and ibuprofen in the Therapeutic Arthritis Research and Gastrointestinal Event Trial (TARGET), cardiovascular outcomes: Randomized controlled trial. *Lancet,* 364: 675–84.
171. La Grenade, L., Kornegay, C. and Graham, D.J. (2000). Using publicly available data to derive background rates when evaluating adverse drug reaction reports (abstract). *Pharmacoepidemiol Drug Saf.*, 9: S70–1.
172. Davis, R.L., Kolczak, M., Lewis, E. *et al.* (2005). Active surveillance of vaccine safety: A system to detect early signs of an adverse event. *Epidemiology*. 16: 336–41.
173. Hawthorne VM, Greaves DA, Beevers DG. Blood pressure in a Scottish town. Br Med J. 1974; 3: 600–3.
174. La Grenade, L., Graham, D.J. and Trontell, A. (2001). Fatal myocarditis with clozapine. *N. Engl J Med.*, 345: 124–5.
175. Frick, P.A., Cohen, L.G. and Rovers, J.P. (1997). Algorithms used in adverse drug reaction reports: A comparative study. *Ann. Pharmacother.*, 31: 164–7.
176. La Grenade, L., Graham, D.J. and Nourjah, P. (2001). Underreporting of hemorrhagic stroke associated with phenylpropanolamine. *JAM, A* 286: 3081.

177. La Grenade, L., Graham, D.J. and Trontell, A. (2001). Fatal myocarditis with clozapine. *N. Engl. J. Med,* 345: 124–5.
178. Friedman, M.A., Woodcock, J., Lumpkin, M.M. *et al.* (1999). The safety of newly approved medicines: Do recent market removals mean there is a problem? *JAMA,* 281: 1728–34.
179. Scott, H.D., Rosenbaum, S.E., Waters, W.J. *et al.* (1987). Rhode Island physicians' recognition and reporting of adverse drug reactions. *R. I. Med. J.,* 70: 311–16.
180. Gurwitz, J.H., Field, T.S., Harrold, L.R. *et al.* (2003). Incidence and preventability of adverse drug reactions among older persons in the ambulatory setting. *JAMA*. 289: 1107–16.
181. Massie, B.M., Berk, M.R., Brozena, S.C. *et al.* (1993). Can further benefit be achieved by adding flosequinan to patients with congestive heart failure who remain symptomatic on diuretic, digoxin, and an angiotensin converting enzyme inhibitor? *Circulation.*, 88: 492–501.
182. Greenblatt, D.J., Haematz, J.S. and Shapiro, L. *et al.* (1991). Sensitivity to triazolam in the elderly'. *N. Engl. J. Med.,* 324: 1691–8.
183. Mukherjee, D., Nissen, S.E. and Topol, E.J. (2001). Risk of cardiovascular events associated with selective COX 2 inhibitors. *JAMA,* 286: 954–9.
184. Larson, A.M., Polson, J. and Fontana, R.J. *et al.* (2005). Acetaminophen–induced acute liver failure: Results of a United States multicenter, prospective study. *Hepatology*. 42: 1364–72.
185. Lindquist, M., Stahl, M., Bate, A. *et al.* (2000). A retrospective evaluation of a data mining approach to aid finding new adverse drug reaction signals in the WHO international database. *Drug Saf.,* 23: 533–42.
186. Crommelin, D., Bermejo, T., Bissig, M., Damiaans, J., Kramer, I., Rambourg, P., Scroccaro, G., Strukelj, B., Tredree, R. and Ronco, C. (2005). Biosimilars, generic versions of the first generation of therapeutic proteins: Do they exist? *Contrib Nephrol.,* 149: 287–294.
187. Blackburn, S.C.F., Ellis, R., George, C.F. and Kirwan, J.R. (1994). The impact and treatment of arthritis in general practice. *Pharmacoepidemiol Drug Saf.,* 3: 123–38.
188. Wiholm, B.E., Olsson, S., Moore, N. and Waller, P. (2000). Spontaneous reporting outside the US. *In*: Strom, B.L. *Ed.*, Pharmacoepidemiology, 3rd edn. New York: Wiley, pp. 175–92.
189. Ostapowicz, G., Fontana, R.J., Schiodt. F.V. *et al.* (2002). Results of a prospective study of acute liver failure at 17 tertiary care centers in the United States. *Ann. Intern. Med.,* 137: 947–54.
190. Szarfman, A., Machado, S.G. and O'Neill, R.T. (2002). Use of screening algorithms and computer systems to efficiently signal higher–than–expected combinations of drugs and events in the US FDA's spontaneous reports database. *Drug Saf.,* 25: 381–92.
191. Kubota, K. (1999). A design for Prescription–Event Monitoring in Japan (J–PEM). *Pharmacoepidemiol Drug Saf.*, 8: 447–56.
192. Greenblatt, D.J., Sellers, E.M. and Shader, R.I. (1982). Drug disposition in old age. *N. Engl. J. Med.,* 306: 1081–8.

193. Conn, H.O. and Poynard, T. (1994). Corticosteroids and peptic ulcer: Meta–analysis of adverse events during steroid therapy. *J. Intern. Med.,* 236: 619–32.
194. Derry, S. and Loke, Y.K. (2000). Risk of gastrointestinal haemorrhage with long–term use of aspirin: Meta analysis. *BMJ,* 321: 1183–7.
195. Hawkey, C.J., Jackson, L., Harper, S.E. *et al.* (2001). Review article: The gastrointestinal safety profile of rofecoxib, a highly selective inhibitor of cyclooxygenase–2, in humans. *Aliment Pharmacol Ther.*, 15: 1–9.
196. Jackson, L.M. and Hawkey, C.J. (2000). COX–2 selective nonsteroidal anti–inflammatory drugs. Do they really offer any advantages? *Drugs,* 59: 1207–16.
197. Urano, W., Taniguchi, A., Yamanaka, H. *et al.* (2002). Polymorphisms in the methylenetetrahydrofolate reductase gene were associated with both the efficacy and the toxicity of methotrexate used for the treatment of rheumatoid arthritis, as evidenced by single locus and haplotype analyses. *Pharmacogenetics,* 12(3): 183–90.
198. Lazarou, J., Pomeranz, B.H. and Corey, P.N. (1998). Incidence of adverse reactions in hospitalized patients. *JAM,* A 279: 1200–5.
199. (2002). American Academy of Pediatrics, Committee on Drugs. Use of drugs not described in the package insert (off–label uses). *Pediatrics.* 110: 181–3.
200. Matthey, P., Wang, P., Finegan, B.A. *et al.* (2000). Rocuronium anaphylaxis and multiple neuromuscular blocking drug sensitivities. *Can. J. Anaesth.,* 47: 890–3.
201. Murdoch, S. and Cohen, A. (2000). Intensive care sedation: A review of current British practice. *Intensive Care Med.,* 26: 922–8.
202. Turner, S., Nunn, A.J., Fielding, K. and Choonara, I. (1999). Adverse drug reactions to unlicensed and off–label drugs on pediatric wards: A prospective study. *Acta Paediatr.,* 88: 965–8.
203. Safety Reporting: Drugs Granted Pediatric Exclusivity, http:// www.fda.gov/ oc/opt/pediatricsafety.html.
204. Dreifuss, F.E., Santalli, N., Langer, D.B., Sweeney, K.P., Moline, K.A. and Menander, K.B. (1987). Valproic acid hepatic fatalities: A retrospective review. *Neurology*. 37: 379–85.
205. Wood, L. and Martinez, C. (2004). The General Practice Research Database: Role in pharmacovigilance. *Drug Saf.,* 27(12): 871–81.
206. Tomeo, C.A., Rich–Edwards, J.W., Michels, K.B. *et al.* (1999). Reproducibility and validity of maternal recall of pregnancy–related events. *Epidemiology,* 10: 774–7.
207. Prieto, L. and Martinez–Frias, M.L. (2000). Response to What kind of controls to use in case control studies of malformed infants: Recall bias versus 'teratogen nonspecificity' bias. *Teratology*. 62: 372–3.
208. Edwards, I.R. (2005). What are the real lessons from Vioxx? *Drug Safety,* 28: 651–8.
209. Kallen, B., Rydhstroem, H. and Aberg, A. (1999). Congenital malformations after the use of inhaled budesonide in early pregnancy. *Obstet Gynecol.*, 93: 392–5.

210. Holmes, L.B, Wyszynski, D.F. and Lieberman, E. (2004). The AED (antiepileptic drug) pregnancy registry: A 6–year experience. *Arch Neurol.*, 61: 673–8.
211. Olsen, J., Czeizel, A., Sorensen, H.T. *et al.* (2002). How do we best detect toxic effects of drugs taken during pregnancy? A Euromap paper. *Drug Saf.,* 25: 21–32.
212. Tabacova, S., Vega, A., McCloskey, C., Kimmel, C.A. (2000). Enalapril exposure during pregnancy: Adverse developmental outcomes reported to FDA. *Teratology*. 61: 520.
213. Selevan, S.G., Kimmel, C.A. and Mendola, P. (2000). Identifying critical windows of exposure for children's health. *Teratology*. 61: 448.
214. Moses–Kolko, E.L., Bogen, D., Perel, J. *et al.* (2005). Neonatal signs after late in utero exposure to serotonin reuptake inhibitors: Literature review and implications for clinical applications. *JAMA*. 293: 2372–83.
215. Honein, M.A., Paulozzi, L.J., Cragan, J.E. and Correa, A. (1999). Evaluation of selected characteristics of pregnancy drug registries. *Teratology*. 60: 356–64.
216. Bombardier, C., Laine, L., Reicin, A. *et al.* (2000). For the VIGOR Study Group. Comparison of upper gastrointestinal toxicity of rofecoxib and naproxen in patients with rheumatoid arthritis. *New England Journal of Medicine*. 343: 1520–8.
217. FDA Arthritis Committee meeting briefing information (2001) February 7 and 8, 2001. http://www.fda.gov/ .
218. Nussmeier, N.A., Whelton, A.A., Brown, M.T. *et al.* (2005). Complications of the COX–2 inhibitors parecoxib and valdecoxib after cardiac surgery. *New England Journal Medicine*. 352: 1081–91.
219. Ray, W.A. and Stein, C.M. (2006). Reform of drug regulation – beyond an independent drug–safety board. *New England Journal Medicine*. 354: 194–201.
220. Bonate, P.L., Kelly, R. and Weir, S. (1998). Drug interactions at the renal level. Implications for drug development. *Clin Pharmacokinet,* 34: 375–405.
221. Cockcroft, D.W. and Gault, M.H. (1976). Prediction of creatinine clearance from serum creatinine. *Nephron*. 16: 31–41.
222. Coleman, J.J. (2004). Drug–induced seizures. *Adverse Drug React Bull*. 227: 871–4.
223. Honig, P.K., Woosley, R.L., Zamani, K. *et al.* (1992). Changes in the pharmacokinetics and electrocardiographic pharmacodynamics of terfenadine with concomitant administration of erythromycin. *Clin. Pharmacol. Ther.,* 52: 231–8.
224. Edoute, Y., Nagachandran, P., Svirski, B. and Ben–Ami, H. (2000). Cardiovascular adverse drug reaction associated with combined beta–adrenergic and calcium entry–blocking agents. *J. Cardiovasc. Pharmacol.,* 35: 556–9.
225. Jackson, S.H.D., Mangoni, A.A. and Batty, G.M. (2004). Optimization of drug prescribing. *Br. J. Clin. Pharmacol.,* 57: 231–6.
226. Pamer, E. and Cresswell, P. (1998). Mechanisms of MHC class I–restricted antigen processing. *Annu. Rev. Immunol.,* 16: 323–58.

227. Park, B.K., Kitteringham, N.R., Maggs, J.L. *et al.* (2005). The role of metabolic activation in drug–induced hepatotoxicity. *Annu. Rev. Pharmacol. Toxicol.,* 45: 177–202.
228. Suzuki, Y., Inagi, R., Aono, T. *et al.* (1998). Human herpesvirus 6 infection as a risk factor for the development of severe drug–induced hypersensitivity syndrome. *Arch. Dermatol.,* 134: 1108–12.
229. Yap, Y.G. and Camm, J. (2000). Risk of torsades de pointes with non–cardiac drugs. *BMJ,* 320: 1158–9.
230. Sibille, M., Deigat, N., Olagnier, V., Vital Durand, D. and Levrat, R. (1992). Adverse events in phase one studies: A study in 430 healthy volunteers. *Eur. J. Clin. Pharmacol.,* 42: 389–93.
231. Kanamaru, M., Nagashima, S., Uematsu, T. and Nakashima, M. (1989). Influence of 7–day hospitalization for Phase I study on the biochemical laboratory tests of healthy volunteers. *Jpn. J. Clin. Pharmacol. Ther.,* 20: 493–503.
232. Wolkenstein, P., Latarget, J., Roujeau, J.C. *et al.* (1998). Randomised comparison of thalidomide versus placebo in toxic epidermal necrolysis. *Lancet,* 352: 1586–9.
233. Chirino, A.J., Ary, M.L. and Marshall, S.A. (2004). Minimizing the immunogenicity of protein therapeutics. *Drug Discov. Today,* 9: 82–90.
234. Knowles, S.R., Uetrecht, J. and Shear, N.H. (2000). Idiosyncratic drug reactions: The reactive metabolite syndromes. *Lancet,* 356: 1587–91.
235. Callot, V., Roujeau, J.C., Bagot, M. *et al.* (1996). Drug–induced pseudolymphoma and hypersensitivity syndrome: Two different clinical entities. *Arch. Dermatol.,* 138: 1315–21.
236. Auquier–Dunant, A., Mockenhaupt, M., Naldi, L. *et al.* (2002). Correlations between clinical patterns and causes of erythema multiforme majus, Stevens–Johnson syndrome, and toxic epidermal necrolysis: Results of an international prospective study. *Arch Dermatol,* 138: 1019–24.
237. Hunkeler, E.M., Fireman, B., Lee, J. *et al.* (2005). Trends in use of antidepressants, lithium and anticonvulsants in youth: 1994–2003. *Journal of Child and Adolescent Psychopharmacology*. 15: 26–37.
238. Murray, M.L., de Vries, C.S. and Wong, I.C.K. (2004). A drug utilisation study. of antidepressants in children and adolescents using the General Practice Research Database. *Archives of Disease in Childhood,* 89: 1098–102.
239. Simon, G.E., Savarino, J., Operskalski, B. and Wang, P.S. (2006). Suicide risk during antidepressant treatment. *American Journal of Psychiatry*. 163: 41–7.
240. Mann, J.J., Emslie, G., Baldessarini, R.J. *et al.* (2006). ACNP task force report on SSRIs and suicidal behavior in youth. *Neuropsychopharmacology*. 31: 473–92.
241. Martinez, C., Rietbrock, S., Wise, J. *et al.* (2005). Antidepressant treatment and the risk of fatal and non fatal self harm in first episode depression: Nested case–control study. *British Medical Journal,* 330: 389–93.
242. Lindquist, M., Edwards, I.R., Bate, A. *et al.* (1999). From association to alert – a revised approach to international signal analysis. *Pharmacoepidemiol and Drug Saf.*, 8: S15–S25.

243. Coulter, D.M., Bate, A., Meyboom, R.H. *et al.* (2001). Antipsychotic drugs and heart muscle disorder in international pharmacovigilance: Data mining study. *BMJ,* 322: 1207–9.
244. Kubota, K., Koide, D. and Hirai, T. (2004). Comparison of data mining methodologies using Japanese spontaneous reports. *Pharmacoepidemiol and Drug Saf.*, 13: 387–94.
245. Bate, A., Edwards, I.R., Lindquist, M. *et al.* (2003). Correspondence: The authors' reply. Violation of homogeneity: A methodological issue in the use of data mining tools. *Drug Saf.,* 26: 363–6.
246. Orre, R., Bate, A., Norén, G.N. *et al.* (2005). A Bayesian recurrent neural network approach for finding dependencies in large incomplete data sets. *International Journal of Neural Systems*. 15: 207–22.
247. Ståhl, M., Lindquist, M., Edwards, I.R. *et al.* (2004). Introducing triage logic as a new strategy for the detection of signals in the WHO Drug Monitoring Database. *Pharmacoepidemiol Drug Saf.*, 13: 355–63.
248. Clark, D.W.J., Donnelly, E., Coulter, D.M. *et al.* (2004). Linking pharmacovigilance with pharmacogenetics. *Drug Saf.*, 7(15): 1171–84.
249. Elliman, D. and Bedford, H. (2001). MMR vaccine: The continuing saga. *BMJ*, 322: 183–4.
250. Fine, K.D. and Schiller, L.R. (1999). AGA technical review on the evaluation and management of chronic diarrhea. *Gastroenterology,* 116: 1464–86.
251. Hawkey, C.J., Jackson, L., Harper, S.E. *et al.* (2001). Review article: The gastrointestinal safety profile of rofecoxib, a highly selective inhibitor of cyclooxygenase–2, in humans. *Aliment Pharmacol Ther.,* 15: 1–9.
252. Patja, A., Davidkin, I., Kurki, T. *et al.* (2009). Serious adverse events after measles–mumps–rubella vaccination during a fourteen–year prospective follow–up. *Pediatr Infect Dis J.*, 19: 1127–34.
253. Locke, G.R., Pemberton, J.H. and Phillips, S.F. (2000). AGA technical review on constipation. *Gastroenterology,* 119: 1766–78.
254. Quigley, E.M.M., Hasler, W.L. and Parkman, H.P. (2001). AGA technical review on nausea and vomiting. *Gastroenterology*, 120: 263–86.
255. Dettling, M., Schaub, R.T., Mueller–Oerlinghausen, B. *et al.* (2001). Further evidence of human leukocyte antigenencoded susceptibility to clozapine–induced agranulocytosis independent of ancestry. *Pharmacogenetics.* 11(2): 135–41.
256. Locatelli, F., Aljama, P., Barany, P. *et al.* (2004). Erythropoiesisstimulating agents and antibody mediated pure red–cell aplasia: Where are we now and where do we go from here? *Nephrol. Dial Transplant,* 19: 288–93.
257. Schellekens, H. (2004). Erythropoietic proteins and antibody–mediated pure red cell aplasia: A potential role for micelles. *Nephrol Dial Transplant.* 19: 2422.
258. Autret–Leca, E., Souda–Grimaldi, L., Jonville–Bera, A.P. and Beau–Salinas, F. (2006). Pharmacovigilance of vaccines. *Arch. Pediatr.,* 13: 175–180.
259. Hartung, H.P., Munschauer, F. III, and Schellekens, H. (2005). Significance of neutralizing antibodies to interferon beta during treatment of multiple sclerosis: Expert opinions based on the Proceedings of an International Consensus Conference. *Eur. J. Neurol.,* 12: 588–601.

260. Schellekens, H. (2002). Bioequivalence and the immunogenicity of biopharmaceuticals. *Nat. Rev. Drug Discov.,* 1: 457–462.
261. Ståhl, M., Lindquist, M., Edwards, I.R. *et al.* (2004). Introducing triage logic as a new strategy for the detection of signals in the WHO Drug Monitoring Database. *Pharmacoepidemiol Drug Saf.,* 13: 355–63.
262. Naranjo, C.A. and Lanctôt, K.L. (1991). Microcomputer assisted Bayesian differential diagnosis of severe adverse reactions to new drugs. A 4–year experience. *Drug Information Journal,* 25: 243–50.
263. Lindquist, M., Ståhl, M., Bate, A. *et al.* (2000). A retrospective evaluation of a data mining approach to aid finding new adverse drug reaction signals in the WHO international database. *Drug Saf.,* 23: 533–42.

Glossary of Acronyms

1. ADME : Absorption, Distribution, Metabolism and Excretion
2. ADROIT : Adverse Drug Reaction Online Information Tracking
3. ADRs : Adverse Drug Reactions
4. AE : Adverse Event
5. AERSs : Adverse Event Reporting Systems
6. API : Active Pharmaceutical Ingredient
7. AR : Adverse Reaction
8. BPCA : Best Pharmaceuticals for Children Act
9. BSR : Summary Bridging Report
10. CCDS : Company Core Data Sheet
11. CCSI : Company Core Safety Information
12. CDSCO : Central Drugs Standard Control Organization
13. CHMP : Committee for Medicinal Products for Human Use
14. CIB : Clinical Investigator's Brochure
15. CIOMS : Council for International Organisations of Medical Sciences
16. CRMs : Chemically Reactive Metabolites
17. CSI : Core Clinical Safety Information
18. DLP : Data Lock Point
19. DSRU : Drug Safety Research Unit
20. DTAB : Drug Technical Advisory Board
21. EBD : European Birth Date
22. EMEA : European Medicines Evaluation Agency
23. EMR : Electronic medical records
24. ESOP : European Society of Pharmacovigilance
25. FDA : Food and Drug Administration
26. FDAMA : Food and Drug administration Modernization Act
27. FDCA : Food, Drug and Cosmetic Act
28. FFDA : Federal Food, Drug and Cosmetic Act
29. GPRD : General Practice Research Database
30. HAI : Health Action International
31. HCP : Health Care Professional
32. HLGT : High Level Group Terms
33. HLT : High Level Terms

34. HTA : Health Technology Assessment
35. IB : Investigation Brochure
36. IBD : International Birth Date
37. ICD9 : International Classification of Diseases
38. ICD9–CM : International Classification of Diseases and its Clinical Modification
39. ICH : International Conference on Harmonization
40. INN : International Non-proprietary Name
41. IRPs : International Reference Prices
42. ISPE : International Society of Pharmacoepidemiology
43. LLT : Level Term
44. MAH : Manufacturing Authorisation Holder
45. MEDDRA : Medicial Dictionary for (Medicines) Drug Regulatory Affairs
46. MedDRA : Medicial Dictionary for (Medicines) Regulatory activities
47. MHRA : Medicines and Healthcare products Regulatory Agency
48. MIMS : Monthly Index of Medical Specialties
49. NCAs : National Competent Authorities
50. NCE : New Chemical Entity
51. NHS : National Health Service
52. OTC : Over the Counter
53. PASS : Post–Authorisation Safety Studies
54. PDUFA : Prescription Drug User Fee Act
55. PEMS : Prescription Event Monitoring System
56. PMS : Post–Marketing Surveillance
57. PPA : Prescription Pricing Authority
58. PREA : Pediatric Research Equity Act
59. PSUR : Periodic Updates Safety Report
60. PT : Preferred Term
61. RMP : Risk Management Plan
62. SAE : Serious Adverse Event
63. SAR : Serious Adverse Reaction
64. SDM : Safety Data Mining
65. SmPC : Summary of Product Characteristics
66. SOC : System Organ Class
67. SUADR : Serious Unexpected Adverse Drug Reaction
68. SUSARs : Serious Unexpected Suspected Adverse Reactions
69. UAR : Unexpected Adverse Reaction
70. UMC : Uppsala Monitoring Centre
71. UNESCO : United Nations Educational, Scientific and Cultural Organisation
72. WHO : World Health Organization

Subject Index

B

C

D

E

F

G

H

N

O

P

Q

R

S

T

U